AIDS and the Church

Other books by the same authors
Published by The Westminster Press

AIDS, a Manual for Pastoral Care
by Ronald H. Sunderland and Earl E. Shelp

A Biblical Basis for Ministry
edited by Earl E. Shelp and Ronald H. Sunderland

AIDS
and the Church

Earl E. Shelp
and
Ronald H. Sunderland

The Westminster Press
Philadelphia

Book design by Gene Harris

First edition

Published by The Westminster Press®
Philadelphia, Pennsylvania

PRINTED IN THE UNITED STATES OF AMERICA

9 8 7 6 5 4 3 2 1

Library of Congress Cataloging-in-Publication Data

Shelp, Earl E., 1947–
　AIDS and the church.

　Bibliography: p.
　1. AIDS (Disease)—Patients—United States—Pastoral
counseling of. 2. AIDS (Disease)—Religious aspects—
Christianity. I. Sunderland, Ronald, 1929–
II. Title. [DNLM: 1. Acquired Immunodeficiency Syndrome.
2. Religion and Medicine. WD 308 S545a]
BV4460.7.S54 1987　　261.8′321969792　　87-14753
ISBN 0-664-24091-7

To our colleague and friend, Jay Jones, who taught us much about AIDS as a consequence of his diagnosis, and members of the Clergy Consultation on AIDS, Houston, Texas, who have been agents of God's love and grace to people caught in the crisis of AIDS.

May this book soon be of historical interest only.

Contents

Acknowledgments

Authors incur many debts in the process of preparing a book for publication. Some debts are to persons and others to institutions. It is impossible to name each person who has made a contribution to this project. Such a list would include the names of hundreds of people who have been touched personally by AIDS. Considerations of confidentiality and privacy prevent us from identifying these patients, families, lovers, and friends. Nevertheless, their willingness to share their experiences with us and to allow us to share in their struggle enabled us to realize in previously unknown ways that love truly is the litmus test of Christian discipleship. We have learned much from these people. We are deeply grateful for their trust.

The medical, social service, nursing, and administrative staff members at the Institute for Immunological Disorders (IID) also cannot be named individually. These women and men have exhibited a compassion and a competency regarding AIDS that are second to none. Peter W. A. Mansell, M.D., and Sue Cooper, M.S.W., who invited us to be part of the staff at IID, have made this volume possible by involving us in a setting and with people whose preoccupation is relieving suffering caused by AIDS. The Institute for Immunological Disorders has been our laboratory. It has no equal.

Members of the interfaith Clergy Consultation on AIDS, who share the dedication of this book, have done the field-testing of the practical proposals presented here. These ordained and lay people have demonstrated their love in the AIDS crisis by implementing spiritual and hands-on ministries. Mostly without fanfare, they have dedicated themselves to replacing fear and estrangement with compassion and reconciliation. Their work is an inspiration.

Jay Jones also can be named. He shares in the dedication of this volume. Had Jay not been diagnosed with AIDS in 1985, it is doubtful that we would have been moved when we were to commit ourselves to advocating to the church and to society the cause of people with AIDS. We grieve for Jay's suffering, but we are grateful for his life and his contribution to our lives.

J. Robert Nelson, Director of the Institute of Religion, and Baruch Brody, Director of the Center for Ethics, Medicine, and Public Issues, have been supportive of our work on this controversial subject. We appreciate their confidence and encouragement to put our thoughts and experiences into print. Attaining that end, however, would not have been possible without the energetic assistance of Ed DuBose, who helped with research, and Delores Smith and Eleanor Cullick, who prepared typescript. Equally as important is the personal or financial support of each of the following, who should know of our appreciation for their role in this project: Jim Denzler, Don and Helen Jones, Jim Myzk, Father Pat Meister and St. Maximilian Kolbe Catholic Church, Father Adam McClosky and St. Mary Magdalene Catholic Church, Robert Fernandez and the Presbytery of the New Covenant, and Bob Peebles and the Cathedral Church of St. John the Divine.

We wish that AIDS had never appeared, and we pray that a cure soon will be found. But since AIDS is a reality and a cure still seems distant, it is our hope that this volume will help the people of God to respond to this expanding public health crisis in an informed and loving manner.

AIDS and the Church

1
The AIDS Crisis

For people who have not come face-to-face with acquired immune deficiency syndrome (AIDS), it may be little more than a curiosity. The media have announced its appearance, reported its spread, and chronicled the vain efforts to reverse or impede its lethal process. Occasionally the public meets someone with AIDS through a televised or printed snapshot portrayal that exposes the syndrome's destructive effect on people's lives. The public reaction has tended to be one of fear, based on an awareness that the virus that causes AIDS is communicable, and a desire to be protected from infection.

From 1981, when illnesses associated with an underlying immune disorder that subsequently would be named AIDS were first described in the United States, until 1985, when film star Rock Hudson's diagnosis and subsequent death were reported, the public seemed willing to ignore AIDS and to develop a false sense of security with respect to it. This apparent indifference probably was related to the mistaken notion that AIDS was a "gay disease," affecting almost exclusively homosexual males, and to a lesser extent a problem for intravenous drug users, another socially disvalued group. However, when pictures of Rock Hudson, near death, appeared on television screens and in newspapers across the nation, AIDS was suddenly

personalized. A gifted, admired, and familiar entertainer
had been stricken. The private devastation and suffering
of thousands became public. AIDS became more difficult
to ignore. Even President Ronald Reagan, who had made
no public statement whatever about the illness before the
disclosure of Hudson's diagnosis, expressed concern for
people struggling to survive AIDS.[1]

Although Rock Hudson's case may be the best publicized, unfortunately it is only one among an ever-
increasing number. Consider Robert.[2] His personal experience with AIDS began in October 1985, when symptoms
of immune system impairment appeared, and surely will
end before this book is published. As these words are
written early in 1987, Robert, who is twenty-six, lies in a
hospital bed with life-prolonging drugs, fluids, and oxygen
running through lines into his body. Robert's lover of
seven years, James, remains by his bedside except when he
must be away. Robert's mother, two half-sisters, who live
in Houston, and his gay older half-brother, who also has
AIDS and lives in New York City, have been summoned
to the hospital. Robert is estranged from his father, who
deserted his mother when Robert was an infant. In the
company of his loved ones, Robert waits for death to take
away his suffering.

Robert discovered his homosexuality when he was
fifteen. His home was not a happy place. His mother had
remarried four times after his father left, with each union
soon ending in divorce. He moved in with a heterosexual
friend, hoping that his homosexuality would disappear or
at least could be sublimated. He shared his sexual feelings
with a trusted friend, who encouraged him to continue in
his effort to overcome them if his desire to be straight was
"from the heart." If, on the other hand, he was merely
trying to conform to what other people expected of him,
he should carefully consider the wisdom of the effort to
deny his sexuality. Following a year of soul-searching,
Robert accepted his homosexuality, returned home, and
invited a teenage friend to live with him. The two were

sexually intimate. Robert's mother learned that he was gay when Robert told her that he needed to be tested for syphilis because his roommate was being tested. The family generally has been accepting of Robert's sexuality, particularly since his older brother had blazed the trail.

Robert moved out of his mother's house when he met James. For seven years James and Robert lived and worked together as laborers. AIDS was a source of worry for them, as it is for nearly all gay men, but they hoped they would escape it since they had been unfaithful to each other on only a few occasions. However, their hope was dashed by Robert's first symptoms of infection in the fall of 1985. The appearance of Kaposi's sarcoma, a malignancy indicative of AIDS, in January 1986 was not a welcome event, but neither was it unexpected. Chemotherapy for the cancer was begun and showed early signs of success. But as is commonly the case, infections developed in the lungs and central nervous system. These infections were treated successfully, but Robert's cancer progressed despite additional therapies. From April until the end of 1986, Robert's condition gradually and persistently worsened. He grew weak, stopped working, lost weight, and struggled to remain optimistic that he would survive.

His current hospitalization will be his last. Kaposi's sarcoma and pneumonia caused by *Pneumocystis carinii* are draining life from him. Now weighing 93 pounds, as compared to 135 pounds before AIDS, Robert coughs violently, labors to breathe, and doubles over from abdominal pain related to his cancer. His skin is discolored and marked by cancerous lesions on all parts of his body. Robert knows that his situation is precarious. He has asked that there be no efforts to resuscitate him when his heart or lungs stop functioning. Dying seems preferable to the suffering that has become his daily companion.

For most of his life, Robert had little interest in God or religion. However, in June 1985 a friend invited Robert and James to worship with a Christian congregation in Houston that has a large homosexual membership. He enjoyed the experience, liked the people he met, and soon

confessed faith in the Lord. He became an active partici-
pant in the church's worship and social functions. His
concern for people with AIDS led to the formation of a
support group for them in the parish. And when he entered the hospital himself, his church friends filled his
room with cards, flowers, balloons, and other expressions
of their love for him.

During the last six months, Robert has belonged to a
prayer group where prayers for his recovery have been a
constant theme. At first these prayers were appreciated.
He believed God would answer them with healing. But as
his condition deteriorated, and death seemed more likely
to be his fate, Robert became disenchanted with the persistent encouragement from group members that he "get
well." Getting well was beyond his control, and it appeared that God was not going to cure him either. His
body tells him now that death is near. Little will be lost
for him when his life ends.

Christmas Day, 1986, was not a day of celebration. The
small decorated tree and gifts, and the presence of James,
his family, and friends in his hospital room, provided
Robert with little cheer. All his energy was directed toward staying alive. None was available for having a good
time. The encouraging and consoling voices of Robert's
loved ones, though appreciated, sounded hollow. Even the
prayers for healing seemed pointless. Robert said in slow
and slurred speech, "They still pray for me to be healed.
But I know that will not happen. Yet they still pray for
my complete healing." Robert's faith in God's love is
unshaken, and he believes he will be with God after he
dies. His faith is strong, but his body and his will to live
are not. The unrealistic prayers of his friends are no longer
a source of comfort. He never wanted to become this
dependent or to look so bad. With great difficulty he says,
"I am too tired to live."

Robert is one of the over twelve hundred men and
women diagnosed as having AIDS, or AIDS-related complex, or as infected by the AIDS virus, who have been seen

in the treatment program in which we work. Our interest in AIDS began during 1982 when we heard of patients who were being denied compassionate care by some of the clinical personnel working in the hospitals at the Texas Medical Center. Other projects kept us from pursuing AIDS as a research subject or as an opportunity for ministry until March 1985, but then we could avoid it no longer. Jay Jones, Earl Shelp's research assistant, unexpectedly became ill with an infection (disseminated histoplasmosis) that subsequently led to a diagnosis of AIDS. Our awareness of AIDS and our intellectual interest in the expanding epidemic thus became a matter of intense personal concern. Our desire to learn as much as possible about AIDS and its effects on people led us to Peter W. A. Mansell, M.D., Director of the AIDS Treatment Program at the M. D. Anderson Hospital and Tumor Institute in the Texas Medical Center. Dr. Mansell and Sue Cooper, M.S.W., opened the world of AIDS to us as they invited us to be consultants to their program. This program has been succeeded by a joint venture between the hospital, the University of Texas Medical School at Houston, and American Medical International, establishing the Institute for Immunological Disorders, the nation's first and only research and treatment center devoted exclusively to AIDS. We serve on the staff at this facility as ethicist (Shelp) and chaplain (Sunderland).

Our experience with Jay, and now hundreds of other patients, has convinced us that the church is only slowly beginning to meet its obligations in this crisis. Whatever guilt or blame attaches to the delayed response to AIDS by church, clergy, and laity belongs to us as well. Perhaps the people of God, individually and corporately, are as we were with respect to AIDS—aware of it but content to avoid the subject and the people burdened by it until it touched home. Thus this volume is written with an attitude of repentance and with an unapologetic passion for the people whose lives are being disrupted and destroyed. Now that we have learned about and have personally experienced the pain, suffering, degeneration, death, and

grief caused by AIDS, we feel compelled to speak pastor-
ally about the challenge AIDS presents. This is not only
a public health crisis of global magnitude, it is a crisis for
the church. AIDS presents the church with an opportunity to reflect on its identity and its mission. Our integrity
and witness are on the line in our response to the AIDS
crisis in general and to people touched by AIDS in particular. Past failures to be a healing and comforting presence
ought to be confessed and must not be perpetuated. There
is no question about the need for such ministry. The
church's willingness and readiness to meet this need, however, are questionable. The church is reluctant to be in the
forefront, forging a compassionate response to AIDS.
While this is regrettable and inconsistent with the
church's calling, it is not unprecedented.

Cultural Reactions to Infectious Disease

Negative religious and moral attitudes have been part
of the social response to infectious diseases and the people
who suffer them for the past 150 years in the United
States. Charles Rosenberg has chronicled the nation's response to the cholera epidemics in 1832, 1849, and 1866,
for example. Cholera is a devastating disease characterized by diarrhea, acute spasmodic vomiting, painful
cramps, consequent dehydration, cyanosis, and possibly
death within hours or days following the onset of symptoms that appear without warning. Unlike the AIDS
virus, the organism that causes cholera *(Vibrio cholerae)*
is easily spread by any pathway to the digestive tract
(food, water, hands). Also unlike AIDS, cholera claimed
relatively few lives. But like AIDS, according to Rosenberg, "it was novel and terrifying, a crisis demanding a
response in every area of American life and thought."[3]
During the epidemic of 1832, cholera was said by many
Americans to be a scourge of the sinful. "Respectable"
people had little to fear. Only intemperate, dirty people
whose behavior predisposed them to cholera were at risk.
This perception of the link between moral judgment and

vulnerability to disease reflected and reinforced prevailing patterns of thought. Cholera was viewed as a consequence of sin, an inevitable and inescapable judgment of God upon people who violated the laws of God. Cholera was not seen as a public health problem. It was an indication of God's displeasure with the people who contracted the disease.[4]

In the epidemic of 1849, the connection between disease and vice still persisted. Also, the belief endured that disease is an expression of God's judgment upon persons and nations corrupted by materialism and sin. But unlike the cholera epidemic of 1832, the needs of people orphaned or made destitute by the disease were not ignored by private charities and committees of "Christian gentlemen." Food, money, clothing, and other forms of assistance were collected and distributed. Some churches joined with these ad hoc committees of lay people, receiving collections for the sick and impoverished. These compassionate ministries were performed even though the victims of cholera were considered guilty of intemperance, gluttony, lechery, or alcoholism. The sickness or death of a so-called respectable person was considered anomalous and conveniently ignored.[5]

The nation's third epidemic of cholera, in 1866, was explained more in scientific than in moral terms. The theory that cholera was caused by a microorganism transmitted to the water supply in feces and vomit gained credibility but not full acceptance. Personal hygiene, sanitation, disinfection, and quarantine became important ways to control the emerging epidemic. Prayer and fasting, stalwarts of previous battles against cholera, were relied upon less in an era of developing scientific knowledge and increased power to combat infection. Thus, as physicians and public accepted an organic cause for cholera, the hand of God was no longer blamed and the belief that moral failure predisposes people to disease lost influence.[6]

This interaction of religious values and social response to infectious disease has not been restricted to cholera. Allan M. Brandt has shown that this pattern of interpreta-

tion and reaction applies equally, if not more so, to venereal disease.[7] Within the past hundred years in the United
States, it was commonly understood that sexually transmitted diseases, principally gonorrhea and syphilis, were
divine punishment upon persons who willfully broke the
moral code of sexual responsibility. When God is perceived as the dispenser of judgment, then efforts, and the
people who undertake them, to control or eliminate the
alleged punishment come to be regarded as anti-God. And
when science defeats God, according to this reasoning,
with a cure or treatment, God finds a new way to express
displeasure. Evangelist Billy Graham reflected this thinking as recently as 1982: "We have the Pill. We have con-
quered venereal disease with penicillin. But then along
comes Herpes Simplex II. Nature itself lashes back when
we go against God."[8] It is implicit in this view that sexual
restraint and behavior modification, due to fear if not
conscience, are the preferred ways to control and combat
sexually transmitted diseases. A consequence of this view
is that people afflicted with a sexually transmitted disease
suffer doubly: the physical effects of the disease itself and
the psychological effects of being stigmatized.[9]

Scientific and therapeutic efforts are undermined when
this attitude prevails. During the 1930s, people with syphilis were refused admission to hospitals, tacitly affirming
the view that these people were morally tainted and less
deserving of care. Afflicted persons, rather than (and in
some instances in addition to) the etiologic biological organism, became the focus of attack.[10] By controlling the
intemperate individuals seen to be carriers or transmitters
of disease, the welfare of the rest of society could be protected. Respectable moral persons were felt to be safe until
nonsexual means of transmission were discovered. Then
calls for the social isolation of carriers were issued. Nevertheless, the attitude persisted that venereal disease was a
disease that preeminently affected others—other races,
other classes, other ethnic groups. Blame easily was placed
on people different from the accuser. Women were favorite targets, since they were supposed to practice sexual

restraint and to uphold prevailing sexual mores. When controlling prostitutes did not decrease the incidence of disease, the role of "good girls" was acknowledged—men totally escaped responsibility—and a profound change in American sexual morality had to be confronted during the 1930s and 1940s.[11]

Educating the public about the effectiveness of condoms as a means to prevent disease was inhibited because of the Roman Catholic Church's opposition to birth control. Fear of disease and pregnancy, not prophylaxis, was the standard weapon against disease. But fear was not very effective. Venereal disease spread. As more "innocents" (people infected by nonsexual routes) and respectable people (people not in some "other" category) were affected, the stigma of disease lessened. Nevertheless, the notion was not forgotten that the entire community was put at risk because of the moral failures of certain disvalued members.[12]

This general pattern of interpretation and response to gonorrhea and syphilis, both before and after 1932, when a cure was discovered, is echoed in the current discussion about AIDS. Medical, governmental, and public concern tended to be anemic until the probable impact of AIDS on people everywhere began to be recognized. AIDS was initially described as a "gay disease." It was considered appropriate punishment for men who violated natural law. Government funding for research and treatment was opposed by leaders of the religious right. Ronald S. Godwin, an executive of the Moral Majority, stated in June 1983, "What I see is a commitment to spend our tax dollars on research to allow these diseased homosexuals to go back to their perverted practices without any standards of accountability."[13] According to this view, homosexuality, not a virus, causes AIDS; AIDS will be eliminated when homosexual persons are eliminated; homosexual persons, not disease-causing organisms, are a threat to the health of society. AIDS, perhaps the ultimate venereal disease, is portrayed as a disease of sinners, an indication of moral decay.

Moral condemnation and wishes that an organism will
be confined to stigmatized people never have been and are
not now effective means of controlling infection. Scape-
goating certain groups and blaming the victims are equally
ineffective. The link of disease to sin may provide a persuasive explanation to some people, and it may be powerful
psychologically, but it is no magic bullet. It compounds
suffering rather than alleviates it, as the history of society's
response to sexually transmitted diseases shows.

The Response to AIDS

Between 1981 and 1983, few people other than those
who could not or chose not to ignore AIDS expressed
much interest in the syndrome or concern for people suffering with it. AIDS was a story, according to NBC science correspondent J. Robert Bazell, that could not be
told when it first appeared because it was seen as a gay
story.[14] Public disregard for gay men took the form of
indifference to a major emerging threat to public health,
probably to the public's peril. Prejudice toward high-risk
groups (gay men and intravenous drug users) joined with
public fears of contagion to foster hysteria and panic.
People with AIDS were fired from their jobs, evicted from
their apartments, denied medical insurance payments, deserted by friends, and abandoned by family members. Funeral directors refused to handle their bodies. Nurses,
medical technicians, and physicians refused to care for
them. Scientific uncertainty and caution were manipulated by political and moral opportunists to further their
respective agendas. People were told to avoid contact with
stereotyped gay service providers: hairdressers, florists,
designers, waiters. Children with AIDS were sent home
from their schools. Fear, ignorance, and hysteria replaced
apathy as the public became increasingly aware that AIDS
is caused by an infectious organism and that valued as well
as disvalued persons were being stricken.[15]
Even as late as 1985 when the evidence was convincing

to most people that the AIDS virus is not easily transmitted, AIDS and the group most identified with it, gay men, were being used as weapons of political warfare. The mayoral campaign in Houston, Texas, was a prime example of manipulation of prejudice. Incumbent Mayor Kathy Whitmire was challenged by Louie Welch, a former mayor and recently retired president of the Chamber of Commerce. Welch announced a four-point plan to control AIDS, one of which was to "shoot the queers."[16] When this remark was inadvertently broadcast live, his campaign managers boasted that record monetary contributions were received as a result, and pastors in his denomination gave him a standing ovation at their prayer breakfast. (Welch subsequently lost the election, however, in an overwhelming defeat.)

Conservative columnist and White House Director of Communications Patrick Buchanan fanned the flames of AIDS hysteria and homophobia when he wrote in 1985 that the "essence" of homosexual life is "runaway promiscuity," which leads to illness and death. "Call it nature's retribution, God's will, the wages of sin, paying the piper, ecological kickback, whatever phraseology you prefer," Buchanan continued.[17] Buchanan's comments not only misrepresent the lifestyle of the vast majority of homosexual people, they reflect a poor understanding of science, philosophy, and theology. William F. Buckley, Jr., a conservative but less vituperative columnist, also has taken note of the AIDS crisis, proposing universal screening for AIDS. If the "AIDS test" is positive, that person "should be tattooed in the upper forearm, to protect common-needle users, and on the buttocks, to prevent the victimization of other homosexuals." These actions are warranted, according to Buckley, because "our society is generally threatened, and in order to fight AIDS, we need the civil equivalent of universal military training."[18] Like that of his colleague, Buckley's proposed solution is based on incorrect evidence. There is no such thing as an "AIDS test." The test to detect antibodies to the AIDS virus is not

perfect and, when accurate, only indicates antibody level
at the time of the test. It does not detect the AIDS virus,
which infects, whereas the antibody it detects does not.
The test only indicates that a person has been infected. It
is not a diagnostic or prognostic tool. Relying on a single
antibody screen to safeguard the public from inadvertent
infection, as counseled by Buckley, would only provide a
safety net that is full of holes.

Finally, followers of political extremist Lyndon
LaRouche attempted to use fear of AIDS to gather support for and validate his political ambitions. The Prevent
AIDS Now Initiative Committee (PANIC) successfully
placed a proposition on the California ballot in 1986 that,
if passed, could have barred infected people from certain
jobs, mandated reporting infected persons to state health
authorities, and possibly sanctioned quarantining persons
with AIDS or people who are well but infected.[19] Like
Buckley's proposal, PANIC's answer for AIDS would not
provide effective protection and totally disregards the
needs of people who are presently ill or infected. The
proposition was not passed by the citizens of California.

The voters' rejection of PANIC's proposition and Louie
Welch's candidacy and the absence of a serious champion
for the proposals by Buchanan and Buckley could be interpreted to mean that the public is well informed about
AIDS, unwilling to be misled by poor logic and misinfor-
mation. However, polls indicate that many people still
think that AIDS can be spread by casual contact. An *NBC
News/Wall Street Journal* poll conducted in January 1986
reported that about one third of respondents thought the
AIDS virus could be spread by eating food handled by a
person with AIDS, being sneezed on, donating blood, or
sharing a drinking glass.[20] A *Newsweek* poll conducted by
the Gallup Organization in July 1986 found that people
have altered their routines to reduce their chances of contracting AIDS by avoiding places where gay men may be
present.[21] These reports of knowledge and conduct suggest
that the public is not adequately educated about AIDS

and that fear remains a powerful influence on responses to the epidemic.

The voices of religious leaders have been part of the public discussion of AIDS. Jerry Falwell has speculated that AIDS could be God's judgment on homosexual persons and society. His political organization Moral Majority opposed government-funded research to find a cure for what it considered a gay problem.[22] In his *Liberty Report* for April 1987 he stated, "AIDS is a lethal judgment of God on America for endorsing this vulgar, perverted and reprobate lifestyle."[23] On the Old Time Gospel Hour, after saddling the "national media, the national press, [and] the educational system in this country" with responsibility for AIDS, he asserted that the "sexual revolution" is being brought to an end by "God Almighty." He stated, "They [male homosexuals] are scared to walk near one of their kind right now. And what we [preachers] have been unable to do with our preaching, a God who hates sin has stopped dead in its tracks by saying do it and die. Do it and die."[24]

Less condemning and more compassionate religious views have been voiced. We were among the first to discuss the issues that AIDS presents to the church in a national ecumenical journal.[25] Eileen Flynn similarly called Catholics to stand with, console, and care for people with AIDS.[26] Bishop William E. Swing, Episcopal Diocese of California, has commented:

> When I read about Jesus Christ in Scriptures and try to understand something of the mind of God, I cannot identify even one occasion where he pictures his Father as occasionally becoming displeased and then hurling epidemics on nations. Especially in relation to sexual matters! Rather than hurling wrath when dealing with an adulteress, Jesus said, "Whoever is without sin, cast the first stone." ... Thus I do not believe in the God who becomes displeased and decides to show his anger by murdering large numbers of people, or in this case homosexual people.[27]

Archbishop John R. Quinn, Roman Catholic Archdiocese of San Francisco, wrote:

> The Christian—the church—must not contribute to breaking the spirit of the sick and weakening their faith by harshness. . . . The presence of the church must be a presence of hope and grace, of healing and reconciliation, of love and perseverance to the end. . . . [AIDS] is a human disease. It affects everyone and it tests the quality of our faith and of our family and community relationships. Persons with AIDS and ARC are our brothers and sisters, members of our parishes. . . . "As disciples of Jesus who healed the sick and is Himself the compassion of God among us, we, too, must show our compassion to our brothers and sisters who are suffering."[28]

Similarly, Roman Catholic conservative Cardinal John J. O'Connor committed the Archdiocese of New York "to do its best to minister to every person who is ill, of whatever disorder, because of our commitment to the belief that *every* person is made in the Image and Likeness of God."[29]

Christian denominations have adopted resolutions and issued statements regarding the church's witness in the AIDS crisis. The first resolution by a church body was adopted in June 1983 by the Fourteenth General Synod of the United Church of Christ. The resolution took note of the slow and meager response of government to a rapidly spreading epidemic and foresaw that AIDS "constitutes a threat to the health of all Americans and to the entire human population worldwide." Through the resolution, the United Church of Christ declared, in part, "its compassionate concern and support for all who are victims of Acquired Immune Deficiency Syndrome and the opportunistic diseases it enables, their lovers, spouses, families, and friends." Parishes were called to support and provide ministries to people touched by AIDS. Finally, the resolution called upon various agencies of government to increase their efforts in combating AIDS' devastating effects.[30]

The 68th General Convention of the Episcopal Church in 1985 adopted a resolution that "recognize[s] with love and compassion the tragic human suffering and loss of life involved in the AIDS epidemic" and "repudiates any and all indiscriminate statements which condemn or reject the victims of AIDS." The Executive Council of the Episcopal Church was charged to develop special intercessory prayers, educational programs, and special ministries. The Presiding Bishop was requested to designate a National Day of Prayer and Healing focused on the AIDS crisis and "to communicate the concerns presented in this resolution to the President of the United States, urging long-term, substantial federal funding for research."[31] The Board of Discipleship of the United Methodist Church adopted a resolution in 1986 stating that, in the midst of AIDS, Christians "are called to accept people as they are, relate them to God's healing grace, and empower them to undertake ministries of compassion and hope." The resolution continued, "We also confess that we as a total church have not always responded lovingly in the midst of this epidemic in part because of deeply held fears and prejudices. We ask God's forgiveness in this regard. We commend to all United Methodist churches this tragic situation as a unique opportunity for ministry and witness."[32]

Oral and written statements embracing reason and compassion have been made by members of other denominations.[33] These expressions of concern and calls to ministry are admirable, though generally issued belatedly. They acknowledge the threat of AIDS, the slow and inadequate response to it, and the obligation of the church to befriend and defend people coping with AIDS. Putting into practice declarations addressing the challenge that AIDS presents to the church tends to be more difficult than making them. Nevertheless, individual Christians and parishes have provided spiritual and hands-on ministries beginning soon after the appearance of this new disease.[34] These ministries have involved commitments of time and money. Some have been provided by individuals, acting alone or with friends. Some have been sponsored by single congregations; others have had diocesan or interfaith sponsorship. In sanctuaries, homes, hospitals, and hospices, some of the people of God have turned toward rather than away from persons caught in the crisis of AIDS. Neither the stigma of AIDS nor the stigma of homosexuality or drug abuse kept them from doing what their faith taught them to do.

The early history of AIDS ministries is difficult to reconstruct in detail, because few reports were published in accessible places. The more recent history of individuals and congregational and denominational ministries is being written in secular and religious magazines, newspapers, and journals. Ministries are proliferating but, unfortunately, not at the same pace as the need. A quantitative gap continues to exist. Verbal confessions of love for a neighbor touched by AIDS have not tended to become acts of love for that same neighbor. The opportunities for ministry that AIDS presents vary among persons and places. A question that must be answered by the faithful is whether and how these opportunities will be met. Moderate voices calling the people of God to loving witness are beginning to be heard and answered. As a result, perhaps the church soon will assume a leadership role in modeling a compassionate, reasoned, and reasonable response to the AIDS crisis. Perhaps love will replace fear among the faithful and the public. Perhaps hope will replace despair among the sick and their loved ones. Perhaps AIDS will become an opportunity for reconciliation rather than estrangement.

AIDS is the latest of several diseases to evoke fear among people and to challenge the church to reflect on its identity and mission. Fear about AIDS is being reduced by a growing body of scientific and medical evidence. Failures in discipleship can be confessed and corrected. Calls to ministry can be answered with a witness that is obedient to and honors the Lord. It has not been easy to have a clear perception of what should be an appropriate response to AIDS. The disease itself initially was shrouded in mystery. Scientists were not sure whether it might disappear as suddenly as it had appeared. Thus in this respect the church's slow response may be understandable. But now it is clear that, although the virus is not easily communicated, AIDS is a growing, global health crisis that has an unprecedented potential for destroying lives. In the face of such an obvious crisis, God's people must begin now to mobilize, to design, and to implement a variety of sustaining ministries in the name of the Lord who commanded his people to love one another.

The religious voices that condemn people touched by AIDS and counsel that the church abdicate its duty toward them are beginning to fade. People are listening less to those who use scripture as an instrument of repression. The arguments and conclusions that initially led to harsh, uncaring interpretations of AIDS are increasingly recognized as flawed, now that the epidemic increasingly affects other than gay people in this country and its global demographics are becoming known. The true liberating, healing witness of the Bible is being heard and followed as the faithful perceive the magnitude of human suffering wrought by AIDS and their obligations with respect to it. Education about AIDS and a broadening experience with it are destroying the myths, stereotypes, and prejudices that have inhibited an empathetic and supportive response. This volume is a contribution to a corrective educational effort. It provides biblical, theological, and ecclesiastical analyses that articulate and justify a redemptive interpretation of AIDS and proposes for God's people a compassionate response to all AIDS victims.

Chapter 2 provides a scientific medical, epidemiological, and psychosocial overview of AIDS and its effects on people. Chapter 3 examines God's role in illness and the responsibilities of the faithful to sick people, concluding that AIDS is not God's retribution on any person or any group of persons and that God's people have a duty to care for the sick, regardless of the nature of the sickness or the means by which people become ill. Chapter 4 advances and defends the claim that people touched by AIDS are contemporary instances of the "poor" toward whom the people of God have a special mission. This mission is expressed in two ways: (1) by advocating the cause of the "AIDS population" where their voices are too weak to be heard and (2) by supporting them with direct, sustaining ministries. The analysis turns from interpretation to application in chapter 5, where descriptive proposals for AIDS ministries are provided. The volume concludes in chapter 6 with a summary defense of the claim that God's people have no option in the AIDS crisis but to design and implement a compassionate, healing, and prophetic ministry that sets an example for all of society to follow.

2
The AIDS Epidemic

When the clinical condition eventually named acquired immune deficiency syndrome, or AIDS, was first described in the United States during 1981, few people foresaw the magnitude of the sickness and death that were to come. Neither was the difficulty of discovering the cause of this new phenomenon and of finding a cure foreseen. The initial reports of unusual infections and malignancies among male homosexuals generally were considered medical curiosities, not preliminary evidence of the destructive potential of a new virus being spread globally. Almost totally without public attention or concern, a new chapter in the history of medicine and public health had begun. No one knows yet when or how it will end. Until then, however, men, women, and children around the world face an epidemic with an unprecedented deadly potential.

AIDS is less mysterious today than it was in 1981. Much has been learned about the AIDS virus and its effects on the human body. Much more will have to be learned before the physical destruction it causes can be stopped. Moreover, the public needs to learn more about AIDS in order to transform ignorance into knowledge and indifference into compassion. The church can and should take a leadership role by becoming educated about AIDS and modeling a caring response toward people touched by it. Educating the church about AIDS is the focus of this chapter.

Early Observations and Theories
and the Discovery of HIV

Beginning in June 1981, physicians in New York City and San Francisco reported the appearance of *Pneumocystis carinii* pneumonia (PCP), other opportunistic infections (infections that result in clinical illness when the immune system is weakened), and a disseminated form of a cancer called Kaposi's sarcoma in apparently previously healthy young gay men. Any one of these diseases would have been unusual in this group, but such a constellation of disorders was unprecedented. Medical scientists and epidemiologists soon realized that these reports were signaling the onset of an apparently new illness in this country. Speculation began immediately about its cause.[1]

Surveys of patients showed that they tended to be sexually active, engaging in practices involving fecal contact and having contact with large numbers of homosexual and bisexual men. This information suggested that perhaps an immunosuppressive substance was being used or an immunosuppressive pathogen was being transmitted from person to person through bodily fluids. Suspicion that the causative agent was immunosuppressive was based on laboratory data indicating an impaired immune system, a system unable to counter infections with an effective defense. This is why infections indicative of AIDS are characterized as opportunistic—the illness is caused by a pathogen that would be controlled or destroyed by a competent immune system. Thus, opportunistic infections take advantage of the immune system's impaired function, resulting in illness where otherwise none would occur.

Researchers tried to explain the observed impaired immune response by studying the immunosuppressive effects of a commonly used inhalant (amyl and butyl nitrite, or "poppers") and of human semen absorbed into the bloodstream through small tears in the rectum during anal intercourse. These studies and other hypotheses related to lifestyle factors led nowhere. The appearance of AIDS among heterosexual intravenous drug users and heterosexual hemophilia patients using a blood clotting agent (Factor VIII concentrate) suggested that the etiologic agent of AIDS not only was transmitted sexually but also was transmissible by blood or blood products. If the causative agent could be carried by blood, it had to be small enough to escape being removed during the process of preparing Factor VIII. This finding ruled out bacteria and fungi, but not viruses. Consideration was given to Epstein-Barr virus and cytomegalovirus, members of the herpesvirus family, because evidence of these viruses was found in patients. However, neither virus was known to produce illnesses like AIDS, nor does either virus have an affinity for the T_4 cells of the immune system. The T_4 or T helper cell is a white blood cell that has a key role in regulating the body's immune system. Studies indicated that T_4 cells were decreased in quantity and quality in people with this new disease.

The search for the elusive virus continued. Because of what had been learned about it indirectly through patient interviews and laboratory studies, it was determined that the cause of AIDS was transmissible through whole blood, plasma, semen, and Factor VIII. Further, as infants born to women with AIDS developed similar illnesses, scientists concluded that the etiologic agent also had to be transmissible congenitally. The collected evidence suggested that the cause of AIDS was likely to be one of a large group of RNA viruses called retroviruses.

Luc Montagnier, head of the Viral Oncology Unit of the Pasteur Institute in Paris, and his colleagues were the first to isolate the virus that was later shown to be the cause of AIDS. In May 1983, the Paris group isolated a new virus from a patient with unexplained swollen lymph nodes, naming it lymphadenopathy-associated virus (LAV). Similar viruses were isolated from the blood of several AIDS patients, but the French were not very successful in growing the virus, a necessary step in the process of identification.

At the same time that the French were doing their research, Robert C. Gallo and his associates at the National Cancer Institute also were looking for a new retrovirus as the cause of AIDS. Gallo's group reported in May 1984 that they not only had isolated a retrovirus that attacked T_4 cells—designated human T-cell lymphotropic virus III (HTLV-III)—but they also were able to grow the virus in sufficient quantities to warrant concluding that this virus caused AIDS. Comparisons of LAV and HTLV-III showed the two to be variants of the same virus. Thus within three years of the appearance of AIDS in the United States, scientists had found the agent responsible for the destruction of T_4 cells and thus for the many secondary clinical illnesses resulting from this deficit in the immune system. Controversy over the name of the virus resulted in a recommendation that these viruses be officially designated as human immunodeficiency viruses (HIV).[2] This term, as well as the colloquial AIDS virus, will be used here.

The Immune System

Identifying the viral cause of AIDS was only one step in the process of finding a cure. Learning how HIV affects the body's immune system was another step. Fortunately, HIV and AIDS appeared at a time in the history of medicine when the technology to study viruses and the immune system was becoming available. In order to appreciate the destructive potential of HIV, it is helpful to have a basic understanding of the cellular components of the human immune system.

The immune system is a flexible but highly specialized defense mechanism that protects the body from invading microorganisms, destroys infected and malignant cells, and removes debris. The precise mechanism by which these tasks are performed is too intricate and complex to pursue here. (For a highly informative presentation of the immune system, see *National Geographic,* vol. 169, June 1986, pp. 702–735.) The process by which infections are normally controlled, however, can be described in simple terms.

White blood cells (lymphocytes) are central to an immune response. There are two classes of lymphocytes: the B cells, which develop in the bone marrow, and the T cells, which also develop in the bone marrow but mature in the thymus gland. B cells produce potent chemical weapons called antibodies that identify antigens (substances that stimulate the production of antibodies) and aid in their removal or destruction. T cells perform three functions. The killer T cell destroys cancerous cells and body cells that have been invaded by foreign organisms. The T helper cell (T_4), unlike B cells and killer T cells, does not directly confront the enemy, so to speak. It is the commander in chief of the immune system. After being summoned to the site of a foreign organism by the macrophages (frontline troops of the body's defensive army), the T helper cell stimulates the production of killer T cells and B cells to combat the intruder. After an intruder or infection has been defeated, a third type of T cell, the suppressor T cell (T_8), calls off the attack by killer T cells and B cells. Thus, T_4 cells turn on the immune response; macrophages, killer T cells, and B cells are combatants; and T_8 cells turn off the immune response. Following a successful defense, a population of T and B cells persists that "remembers" the invader. Should the invader appear again, the immune response will be accelerated because the enemy is recognized more quickly.

Among the cells that constitute the cellular immune system, the T helper cell has the key role in orchestrating a defense of the body against infections. Without an adequate quantity and quality of T helper cells, the body's defensive forces are ineffectively mobilized, if at all, when challenged. The AIDS virus is able to defeat the body's immune response by preemptively destroying its commander in chief. When the T helper cell is infected by HIV it

nes a factory within which additional HIV is pro-
1. As an HIV-laden cell dies, viruses escape to con-
ther cells with appropriate chemical receptors that
allow entry. The number of T helper cells, which normally
constitute between 60 and 80 percent of the circulating T
cells, can be reduced in AIDS to a level where they become too few to be detected. Thus, as more T helper cells
are infected, harbor replicating virus, die, and release
more virus to attack the remaining competent T helper
cells, the immune system becomes progressively impaired,
rendering the body vulnerable to microorganisms and
physiological processes that otherwise would not result in
clinical illness.

Origin and Transmission of HIV

Identifying the viral cause of AIDS and learning about
the effect of HIV on the body's immune response are
important discoveries. The clinical story of AIDS began
in the United States in 1981, but investigators learned that
the virus did not originate here. The search for its source
led researchers to Africa, where AIDS had been identified
soon after it was recognized in the United States.

Retrospective analyses of stored blood from Africa
show that HIV was present in Kinshasa, Zaire, in 1959.
Studies of banked blood from west and east Africa indicate the presence of HIV in the 1960s and 1970s, whereas
tests of blood from other parts of the world collected
during those decades detect no antibodies to HIV. Thus,
serologic and epidemiologic evidence suggests that HIV
originated in central Africa, and it remains today most
prevalent in the central part of that continent.

In 1985, scientists isolated a retrovirus found in African
green monkeys that resembled HIV. This monkey virus
(simian T-lymphotropic virus III or STLV-III) does not
produce pathology in green monkeys. But the possible link
of STLV-III to HIV became more plausible as variations
or mutated forms of HIV from west Africa were isolated
by French and Swiss scientists. Unlike STLV-III, these

mutated forms of HIV, which resemble STLV-III, do cause immune deficiency in the human host. These discoveries have led Robert Gallo to consider as a plausible hypothesis "that STLV-III somehow entered human beings, initiating a series of mutations that yielded the intermediate viruses before terminating in the fierce pathology of HTLV-III."[3] Epidemiologists speculate that the AIDS virus remained localized in central Africa until the early 1970s, at which time it spread to other parts of Africa. Toward the end of the 1970s it spread to Haiti and may have entered the Americas and Europe from there.

By tracing the origin of HIV to Africa and studying its history there, a major myth about AIDS is revealed to be false. In Africa, AIDS is not linked to homosexual male contact. It affects heterosexual males and females in approximately equal numbers. Thus, AIDS is not a gay disease. Neither is it a drug addict's disease, a hemophiliac disease, or a disease attributable to any particular group of persons. Rather, AIDS is a possible consequence of infection by HIV in any person without regard for any identifying characteristic. HIV aptly has been described as an "equal opportunity virus." Homosexual and heterosexual persons, male and female, white and black, young and old are all equally subject to infection if virus particles or infected cells gain direct access to the bloodstream. Certain practices permit this to happen: anal intercourse (the passive partner is at greater risk), vaginal intercourse (male-to-female and female-to-male transmission have been documented), use of nonsterile needles, receipt of contaminated blood or blood products, and transmission from a mother to her fetus. These are the only proven ways by which the AIDS virus is spread.

It is true that HIV has been isolated in tears and saliva, but only rarely in infected individuals and at levels probably too low to be damaging. It should be noted, as well, that there is no evidence that the virus penetrates the skin, epithelial cells lining the respiratory tract, or mucosa of the digestive tract. Thus, casual contact, coughs, sneezes, and consumption of food prepared by infected persons present no known risk of infection. Transmission by insects is unlikely and has not been demonstrated. There is no risk of infection by donating blood at centers where sterile procedures are used. Though HIV is potent once it enters the body, it is fragile outside the body. Most household detergents, common disinfectants, and moderate heat (158°F for ten minutes) can kill the virus. Studies of health care personnel and families of patients indicate that none have been infected as a result of casual, even daily, contact with infected individuals. Infected blood, semen, and vaginal secretions appear to be the only bodily fluids by which HIV can be transmitted, provided the virus has entry into the bloodstream.

Epidemiology

AIDS is an epidemic more in the sense of the estimated number of people worldwide infected with HIV than in the sense of the number of people with a confirmed diagnosis of AIDS. For example, African countries tend not to have the health services or adequate resources to assess the incidence of infection. The technical equipment may not be available to confirm a diagnosis of opportunistic infections and malignancies and to exclude other causes of immunodeficiency. Finally, diagnostic services for opportunistic infections and for HIV infection are in short supply. Thus it is impossible to determine the actual incidence of AIDS and HIV infection on the continent where they have the longest history. It is clear, however, from available data that in Zaire the incidence of AIDS is approximately 17 cases per 100,000 population, compared to a rate of 6 per 100,000 population in the United States. The experience in Zaire may or may not be representative of other African countries or predictive of the experience in the United States. There are studies indicating that 5 to 10 percent of the population of central Africa may be infected with HIV. If so, millions of people, on a continent largely without effective means to limit the transmission of the AIDS virus, are candidates for AIDS.

In the United States, the number of AIDS diagnoses continues to grow at a rapid rate. In 1986 the Public Health Service (PHS) issued five-year projections for the epidemic. This report estimates that by the end of 1991 the cumulative total of AIDS cases will exceed 270,000, with more than 74,000 occurring in 1991. Of this number, more than 179,000 will have died, with over 54,000 deaths occurring in 1991. These are sobering estimates. They are an even greater cause for concern if, in fact, they underestimate by 20 percent the actual morbidity and mortality attributable to AIDS, as the PHS report admits may be the case. The number of people presently infected with HIV is conservatively estimated at 1.5 million as of June 1986. No one knows how many people will be infected by 1991. Much depends on successful behavior modification and educational programs designed to reduce the spread of the virus. It is likely, however, that at least 25 to 50 percent of HIV-infected people will progress to AIDS within five to ten years following infection.

Homosexual and bisexual men and intravenous drug users in the United States presently constitute about 90 percent of cumulative AIDS cases. It is likely that these groups will continue to be at highest risk for infection and disease because this is where the virus was first established in this country. The proportion of gay and bisexual men with AIDS seems to be decreasing, however, and the proportion of intravenous drug users appears to be growing, probably because it is easier for gay and bisexual men to practice "safe sex" than for IV drug users to alter their behavior. Also, as the AIDS virus penetrates further into the heterosexual population, their numbers are projected to increase from 4 percent of patients in December 1986 to 10 percent in 1991.

The capacity to determine infection was greatly enhanced during 1985 with the approval of a blood-testing process called enzyme-linked immunosorbent assay (ELISA).[4] This relatively simple and inexpensive test was developed to screen donated blood for antibodies to the AIDS virus, thus reducing the risk of infection by transfusion or use of blood products. Although these tests are not 100 percent accurate, they are highly reliable and considered an effective means of protecting the blood supply. The ELISA is also used to determine the infection status of people in clinical settings. The test is not considered to be a diagnostic test or to be predictive of who will ultimately develop clinical illness as a consequence of infection. The test, if positive, only indicates the presence of antibodies to the AIDS virus at a sufficient level to activate the test at the time the tested blood was drawn. If the test is negative, it means that the tested blood does not have a sufficient level of AIDS virus antibodies to activate the test. A person may, nevertheless, be infected. Thus it is recommended that people at high risk for infection be tested every six months if they wish to monitor their infection status. When a person is antibody-positive for the AIDS virus, he or she should be considered infectious and take precautions not to infect others. With the ELISA, it could be possible to determine the actual incidence of infection in the population, but public health authorities have decided against universal testing since the test is not diagnostic or predictive.

AIDS and HIV truly are global concerns. Reports from Great Britain, Europe, Scandinavia, South America, South Pacific countries, the Soviet Union, and Asia indicate the scope of the problem. Perhaps as many as 10 million people in the world presently are infected. Unfortunately, the rising incidence of HIV infection and AIDS is not likely to be reversed in the foreseeable future. Thus disease and death as a consequence of HIV infection are likely to increase at least for the next five to ten years and probably into the twenty-first century.

AIDS and Related Diagnoses

AIDS is the most widely known clinical diagnosis that may follow infection by HIV. It is not generally understood among the public, however, that AIDS is not the most common HIV-related diagnosis. Two additional clinical diagnoses are more common but less publicized: AIDS-related complex (ARC) and lymphadenopathy syndrome (LAS). The most common clinical category, as can be inferred from the above epidemiological data, is either HIV antibody-positive (presence of antibodies to HIV in the blood) or HIV viremia (presence of HIV in the blood). According to the Centers for Disease Control (CDC) surveillance definition, AIDS is an illness characterized by one or more designated cancers or opportunistic infections that are at least moderately indicative of an underlying cellular immunodeficiency for which there is no other known cause than HIV infection and the absence of all other causes of reduced resistance to a particular disease.[5] In other words, a person must test positive for HIV antibodies or virus *and* manifest a designated infection or cancer indicative of AIDS to be diagnosed as having AIDS. Numerous infections—protozoal, helminthic, fungal, bacterial, and viral—meet the inclusion criteria for AIDS, as do two forms of malignancy. Protozoal and helminthic infections include cryptosporidiosis, *pneumocystis carinii* pneumonia, strongyloidiasis, isosporiasis, and toxoplasmosis. Fungal infections include candidiasis, histoplasmosis, and cryptococcosis. Bacterial infections include *Mycobacterium avium* or *intracellularis* and *Mycobacterium kansasii.* Viral infections include cytomegalovirus, herpes simplex virus, and progressive multifocal leukoencephalopathy. The malignancies associated with AIDS include Kaposi's sarcoma, brain lymphoma, small noncleaved lymphoma, and immunoblastic sarcoma.[6] The inclusion criteria for AIDS are subject to revision as more clinical presentations are linked to HIV infection.

A detailed explanation of each of these diseases would not be helpful here. What is important is that each disease, in its own way, exacts a heavy toll on a person whose immune system is permanently compromised. Also, it is common for people with AIDS to have two or more of these conditions active at the same time. AIDS-related infections typically affect the lungs, gastrointestinal system, bone marrow, and central nervous system. Kaposi's sarcoma typically appears first on the skin but in more than 75 percent of patients it spreads to the lymph nodes, lungs, or gastrointestinal tract. The lymphomas in AIDS tend to appear most commonly in the central nervous system, bone marrow, and bowel, but also in other sites.

Some of these diseases are responsive to conventional or experimental treatments. It should be emphasized, however, that recovery does not mean that a particular disease will not reappear later. Many patients have recurring acute episodes of the same disease, or the disease becomes chronic. This phenomenon of multiple, sequential, major acute illnesses, alone or in combination with chronic illnesses typical of AIDS, results in a course that often is unpredictable. Patients may deteriorate gradually or rapidly. Their loss of control over their bodies and lives mirrors, in most instances, the features and rate of their deterioration. About the only predictable aspect of AIDS, given the present state of therapeutics, is that death within two years of initial diagnosis will occur for approximately 80 percent of patients, and within four years for nearly 100 percent.

AIDS-related complex (ARC) is a clinical diagnosis for people who have a variety of chronic symptoms and physical findings associated with HIV infection but which do not satisfy the strict criteria for AIDS established by the Centers for Disease Control. As AIDS was beginning to be understood, physicians hoped that ARC would be a less severe and nonlethal consequence of HIV infection. But experience has shown that ARC illnesses can result in death without the patient's progressing to AIDS. The symptoms of ARC include chronic swollen glands, recurrent fevers, unintentional dramatic weight loss, chronic diarrhea, lethargy, and oral fungal infections. These problems appear manageable, and in many persons they are successfully treated for a long period. However, some patients succumb to the wasting and nonopportunistic infections typical of ARC. It is impossible to be certain of the number of people with ARC or to predict what percentage of ARC patients will develop AIDS. ARC is not a uniform or reportable clinical diagnosis, so no national or international data exist. Physicians estimate, however, that the number of people in the United States with ARC may be 4 to 10 times greater than the number of people with AIDS. Finally, ARC can be debilitating, resulting in patients' becoming dependent upon others for assistance in performing routine tasks.

While the actual number is not known, epidemiologists are certain that people with lymphadenopathy syndrome (LAS) outnumber people with AIDS and ARC. LAS is a condition characterized by persistent (longer than three months) generalized swollen glands that cannot be explained by a current illness or drug use known to cause such symptoms. The number of persons in the United States with LAS may be 10 to 100 times the number of people with AIDS. As with ARC, no one knows how many people with LAS will progress to ARC or AIDS. Further, patients with this early clinical indication of HIV infection may not progress to ARC before progressing to AIDS, if at all. The presence of certain co-factors may influence whether progression occurs and at what rate. These factors are thought to include a prior history of infectious diseases and lifestyle patterns involving poor diet, lack of exercise and rest, unusual stress, and use of alcohol and drugs.

Finally, the largest clinical category of people infected with HIV are those who thus far have no symptoms of infection. Many, if not most, are not even aware that they are infected and, presumably, infectious. As has been indicated, there may be as few as 1.5 million or as many as 3 million people in the United States already infected by HIV. The future for these individuals is unclear. What number will progress to some form of clinical illness is not yet known. Studies of infected individuals over time will help provide this information.

Before we discuss other features of the AIDS epidemic, it is important to take a brief look at the psychiatric and neurologic complications of HIV infection. We saw that HIV has a devastating effect on the immune system by destroying the quantity and effectiveness of a key cell, the T helper cell. HIV infects this cell because it has a chemical receptor on its surface that permits the virus to penetrate it. It should not be overlooked, however, that HIV can invade other cells in the body with appropriate receptors to allow it entry.[7] While it was thought early on that HIV only infected T helper cells in the immune system, further studies have shown that HIV may be able to infect any cell. This means that HIV may be the cause of certain illnesses, as well as creating the conditions in which other organisms may produce illness. This process of HIV-induced illness is seen dramatically in the central nervous system.

HIV was first detected in brain (glial) cells and in spinal cord tissues in 1984. This discovery is significant for several reasons. First, it suggests that HIV may be, more than originally thought, like a family of retrovirus that causes neurological disease in other animals. This means that HIV may be capable of incubating in the body for years, perhaps as long as fifteen years, before symptoms of neurological disease appear. Second, antiviral agents must be able to penetrate the blood–brain barrier in order to be successful. Therapies that only remove the virus from the blood will not be adequate. A cure must also entail removing HIV from brain cells in a way that is nontoxic to brain tissues. Third, neurological impairments related to or caused by HIV will place additional strains on the health care system. This potentially large population eventually could exhibit major physical impairments and severe neurological disabilities that require intensive medical and custodial care.

The psychiatric and neurological complications of HIV infection may range from minor to severe, even lethal.[8] In addition to opportunistic infections and lymphomas of the central nervous system, patients often develop some level of dementia, psychosis-like illnesses, and other neurological syndromes, such as multiple sclerosis. The most common neurological complaints of patients are memory loss, confusion, agitation, peripheral neuropathies, seizures, and decreased coordination. In about 10 percent of patients, neurological complaints are the first symptom of HIV infection. Postmortem examinations of patients have confirmed the extent of HIV neurological involvement. About 90 percent of patients have demonstrable abnormalities of the nervous system. These data underscore the extensive, devastating potential of HIV to infected individuals and those involved in their care.

Psychosocial Aspects and the Economic Impact of AIDS

The physical and mental manifestations of HIV infection tend to be most severe and debilitating with full-blown AIDS. The debility and dependency that accompany the progression of disease in the body can have a correspondingly severe effect on a patient's family and friends and on the public at large. In some instances, the psychosocial consequences of an AIDS or AIDS-related diagnosis can be as devastating as the disease itself. The discussion of these matters will be divided into four parts, with each part focusing on different groups touched by the AIDS epidemic.

Patients, Families, and Friends

When a person is told by a physician that she or he has AIDS, ARC, or LAS, a series of adjustments are set in motion, adjustments that affect every aspect of a patient's life. Family relationships, romantic involvements, friendships, and occupational ties suddenly are cast in a new light. Perspectives and priorities may change. Decisions about oneself and plans for the future require reexamination. Obviously these matters generally appear more urgent to people with AIDS and ARC than to people with LAS or HIV-positive diagnoses. Since AIDS and ARC in the United States are most prevalent among young adults, who normally are not anticipating debility and death, their diagnosis tends to set in motion a transition from being vigorous to being debilitated, symptom-ridden, and probably dying, often within months. This abrupt change in status and self-perception requires a massive adjustment. It tends to be easier for patients who were psychologically stable before the diagnosis and who have loyal and cohesive support systems.

Patients frequently use the defense mechanism of denial to exercise control over how and when they will face the matter of their own mortality. Denial tends to be less effective among AIDS patients because the lethal character of their diagnosis is reinforced by frequent media reports, discouraging medical developments, and the deaths of friends. It is hard to be hopeful about the future. The sense of insecurity (because palliative and curative treatments are unavailable) is heightened by financial, career, and relational limitations common to young adults. Fears about infecting others and guilt about transmitting HIV to past sexual partners also may have a role in the adjustment process. IV drug users and gay and bisexual men who have kept their sexuality secret may have to disclose to family and friends this feature of their lives, not knowing for certain how others will respond. The threat of condemnation and abandonment intensifies the distress of patients in these situations.

Diminished self-esteem, depression, and suicidal thoughts are common. The stigma attached to AIDS; concern about a loss of autonomy due to weakness, blindness, and mental deficits; social rebuke and rejection; and discrimination in work, housing, insurance, and social services contribute to the psychological trauma of the diagnosis. Having watched a lover or friend struggle against the dignity-robbing effects of AIDS, patients tend to approach their illness with dread, fearful of the disfigurement, debilitation, wasting, and death that may already be all too familiar. The appearance of Kaposi sarcoma lesions on visible parts of the body tends to provoke anger, anxiety, and, for some, resignation to a self-imposed, if not externally imposed, isolation. Published calls for quarantine and universal criminalization of homosexuality, abandonment or reports of abandonment, and fears that no one will handle one's corpse in a respectful manner compound the anxiety that patients experience about their present and future state. Living alone, perhaps abandoned by friends and estranged from family, patients worry about what will happen when they are unable to care for themselves. Nursing homes and hospices may not be available because of a lack of funds or because the doors are not open to them. Finally, knowing that they are infectious but still desiring intimate contact to meet a variety of psychological and emotional needs can create distress and anxiety. Feeling unattractive and untouchable, patients have a significant need for affirmation and affection, which often can be shown by a simple pat on the shoulder, a kind word, or a hug.

Ironically, patients with ARC who progress to AIDS or patients with symptoms of HIV infection but no diagnosis are sometimes relieved when told they have AIDS or ARC. Some of the uncertainty of their condition is removed and their future seems clearer, even if not desirable. Knowing about their status may prompt them to move beyond denial and to cope constructively with their situation. Many begin to put their affairs in order, to plan for their funeral or memorial service, to endeavor to reestablish relationships with people important to them but from whom they are estranged, and to work at enjoying time spent with friends. Other patients become preoccupied with their bodies, at times becoming hypochondriacal. Some who discover that they are infected may adopt healthier lifestyles and practice "safe sex." Others may deny the threat and change nothing or become fatalistic.

The psychosocial aspects of an AIDS or related diagnosis for families are in some ways unique. Many families must deal with the same fears and anxieties about AIDS that the general public confronts. In addition, they may have to respond to disclosures regarding the patient's lifestyle and the resulting strain on relationships. Family members, too, may feel stigmatized and isolated because of their relationship to a person with AIDS, who also may be homosexual or bisexual or an IV drug user. Fears of criticism, ostracism, and embarrassment may prevent families from sharing their burden with others and, as a consequence, deny them the support that otherwise would be provided if the family member's illness was other than AIDS-related.

Families may be angry, feeling that the patient has been irresponsible or sinful and has unnecessarily burdened them. Prejudice against gay and bisexual men suddenly may be directed toward a loved one, threatening the relationship and generating internal conflicts in family members who are not understanding or sympathetic. Ambivalence toward a patient's friends or lover may be an additional source of stress. In particular, family disapproval or rejection of a lover may lead a gay patient to feel that he has to choose between his lover and his family at a time when he needs the loving support and affirmation of all people important to him.

The threat of death carried by AIDS means disruption of the life plans of both patients and families. Parental concerns for the welfare of a child whose death is imminent involve concerns for themselves as well. They mourn the anticipated and actual death. They also grieve the loss of the potential security which that child represented to their old age. Parents frequently say "This isn't natural" or "This isn't the way it's supposed to be." Children are to bury parents, rather than parents burying children. Death vigils may be tense because family members are afraid to hold or kiss their dying loved one. Although a spoken goodbye may be sufficient for some family members, a goodbye that forgoes physical contact may be an occasion for remorse and guilt later. Another complication in family relationships before and after death may develop if the patient has attempted to protect family members by not disclosing the true diagnosis or has allowed the truth to be told too late for meaningful conversations to take place. Family members may feel they have not been trusted and may search to identify where they "failed" the patient. Feelings of rejection, neglect, and abandonment are not uncommon in these situations. Feelings of guilt may develop if a family fears to take the patient home to die because friends and neighbors would learn the truth. And finally, the healing process of bereavement may be frustrated because the usual support from friends and family may be forgone or not available.

Lovers of gay men with AIDS may be a source of conflict with families, if the relationship between the two men is difficult to accept. Families may not accept the lover as a person whose significance to the patient is comparable to a spouse in heterosexual marriage. The stresses typically associated with situations of serious illness may be increased by tensions related to a gay relationship. In addition, a gay patient may legally empower his lover to make decisions about treatment during periods of the patient's incompetence, and families may resent being displaced in this fashion. Issues of control and dissatisfaction with one's sense of emotional importance to the patient can become points of contention between lover, patient, and family.

Lovers tend to have emotional and psychological reactions to their loved one's illness comparable to that experienced by heterosexual spouses. These include anger, grief, and fear. Chronic illness, debility, and premature death are not within the normal expectations of young adults. The stresses imposed on the relationship create needs for support and understanding. The burden of care can be exhausting, physically and emotionally. Plans, dreams, and hopes that will not be fulfilled become sources of grief. The situation at home may be unknown to family and co-workers. For example, lies and excuses explaining exhaustion, irritability, and poor performance may not be satisfactory to an employer. Similarly, absence from work may be difficult to explain without disclosing personal information that could place one's employment in jeopardy. Finally, when death occurs co-workers may be denied the opportunity to be supportive, and the grieving lover may not be excused from daily activities to mourn.

Friends of people with AIDS have many of the same

feelings and reactions as families and lovers. At times friends respond by avoiding the person with an HIV infection, especially if AIDS is diagnosed. In other situations, friends remain loyal, understanding, supportive, and compassionate. People in high-risk groups, such as gay men, may have experienced the death of many friends. Chronic grief is not an uncommon phenomenon. The cumulative loss and pain can become so intense that they seek to avoid any future hurt by disengaging from sick friends. This response may not be callous but rather self-protective. Gay men have said they feel like soldiers watching the rest of their platoon fall in battle one after another.

Health Care Personnel

Because people with HIV infection, especially AIDS and ARC, frequently require medical attention and hospitalization, bonding often occurs with health care personnel. This takes place in both directions, patient to personnel and personnel to patient. Watching patients deteriorate and die in their prime is emotionally draining. There are no major victories in AIDS treatment at present, only minor ones. This situation is discomforting to professionals accustomed to cures, palliation, or remission. Chronic grief is common, and so is physical exhaustion. AIDS patients during acute illnesses tend to require frequent therapeutic interventions and diagnostic procedures. The needs of AIDS patients can seem all-consuming, especially when resources are limited and the needs for care are extensive. Finally, communicating with a patient can be complicated by a patient's neurological condition. Informing a patient about his or her status, explaining options, and responding to questions can be time consuming, especially if a physician treats many AIDS patients. The time required to provide emotional support to patients, families, and friends places even greater demands on the time and energy of health care personnel. Prejudice toward at-risk groups and fear for personal safety may lessen the quality and character of care provided by personnel who serve AIDS patients involuntarily—nurses, resident physicians, and technicians. Some personnel feel ambivalent about their work with these patients, torn between a sense of professional duty toward the sick and negative feelings about conduct related to HIV infection. Finally, health care personnel may be isolated by peers and friends. Colleagues and friends may not value the investment in people with HIV-related diagnoses. Subtle and overt expressions of disapproval of one's professional and moral sense of duty may generate doubts about the worthiness of one's work and ambivalence toward the population served.

Members of High-Risk Groups

We have already noted the prospect for chronic grief among members of high-risk groups. Beyond this, however, fear about one's own well-being and future may be dominant concerns. Each cough or skin blemish may be seen as an omen of worse things to come. Common illnesses become occasions of uncommon concern. Gay and bisexual men often change their behavior patterns in order to reduce risks. Sexual abstinence is less common but not unknown. A person may worry that an infected partner may not disclose this fact, if known. Thus, every partner, if one is to act prudently, is perceived as a potential threat, a situation that undermines trust and mutuality. These threats to personal and community identity are heightened by political efforts to further oppress homosexual men and women.

Intravenous drug users may feel even more neglected and abused as a group than gay and bisexual men. Apart from campaigns to stop drug sales, politicians seem uninterested in individual rehabilitation programs or social programs designed to break the connection between unemployment and poverty and drug use. The belief that no one cares about these people and the health crisis they face with AIDS may not be unfounded. Drug users do not have an organized political lobby in society or in churches to advocate their cause, as does the homosexual population at high risk for AIDS. And drug users tend not to vote or exercise much economic power. Thus this high-risk group may feel even greater despair and hopelessness as HIV spreads from one person to another whenever a needle is shared. Proposals to provide sterile needles to this population deserve careful consideration as one means to help limit the unceasing advance of AIDS.

The Public at Large

The public justifiably is concerned about the present and potential impact of AIDS. Apart from reports of fearful reactions to people with AIDS, the syndrome generally was a matter of marginal concern until it was perceived as a threat to heterosexual people who are not IV drug users. The voices of scientists calling attention to the growing magnitude of the epidemic finally are being heard. Yet the unavailability of absolute answers to many questions regarding transmission of HIV and conflicting interpretations of available data generate confusion. This confusion seems to impede a comprehensive, informed, and coordinated response to AIDS, in terms of research, treatment, and prevention.

Public education activities have been limited because the audience has tended not to be receptive. In addition, informing people about the means of HIV infection requires discussing sexuality and IV drug use, and both subjects are potentially explosive. Finally, prophylactics that protect people from infection during heterosexual intercourse—condoms—are also contraceptive, another morally controversial topic to some people. The dilemma the public faces ought not be underestimated. Massive educational programs aimed at prevention are imperative. Yet the goal of prevention may be at odds with the moral values of certain segments of the population. How this dilemma will be resolved is still uncertain.

Another area of public concern involves the response to people presently suffering with AIDS and related diagnoses. When the extent of suffering is made known, even if the ones suffering are not highly regarded, people tend to be moved to compassion. Informing the public of this situation without unnecessarily exposing the wasting bodies and minds of people with AIDS may be difficult. Verbal descriptions are not as compelling as personal testimonies and visual images. But once moved to compassion, the public must consider the claims of the AIDS population for care in relation to the claims of people struggling with other illnesses. Profound issues of distributive justice, as well as mercy, warrant consideration. Here the economic impact of AIDS becomes pointedly relevant.

Economic Impact of AIDS

Early estimates of the dollar and economic costs of AIDS in the United States were ominous. Analyses of the first 10,000 cases of AIDS indicated that hospitalization costs would be about $1.4 billion and the economic loss from future earnings due to premature death would be $4.6 billion.[9] These totals do not reflect expenditures for testing, counseling, blood screening, monitoring asymptomatic persons, and treating people with ARC and LAS. More recent studies indicate that the total lifetime hospitalization costs per AIDS patient range between $42,000 and $50,000. This estimate is decreased from earlier estimates of $150,000 per patient. Although this reduction is encouraging, it does not mean that the total cost of AIDS is decreasing. An increasing AIDS population means that total costs are likely to increase. The Public Health Service estimates that direct costs to care for people with AIDS in 1991 will grow to between $8 and $11 billion, constituting 1.2 to 2.4 percent of the expected total personal health care expenditures in the United States.[10] It should be noted that these more recent estimates of current and projected expenditures do not account for lost earnings, as did the early report. Nor do they reflect expenditures for ARC, LAS, testing, screening, and monitoring. Finally, neither the early nor the more recent analyses measure the intan-

gible costs of pain, suffering, adverse effects on relationship, and social stigmatization. Clearly, the impact of HIV
on the demand for hospital beds, professional services,
drugs, supportive services, and hospice care is already
significant and will grow. Public education programs and
social programs aimed at risk reduction will add to the
economic burden.

This selected overview of the psychosocial aspects and
economic impact of AIDS only begins to portray the ripple effect of HIV. The picture of pain, suffering, and death
truly is overwhelming when the experience in the United
States is extended to include the rest of the world. There
may be no other microorganism in history to equal the
sweeping destructive effect of HIV.

Prevention and Prospect for Treatment

It should be obvious that education to help reduce risks
is at present the best defense against HIV. But several
questions must be answered before these efforts can be
expected to succeed. What should be the content of public
education? What are the aims of public education? Who
needs education? Who should do the educating? How
should educational programs be funded and evaluated?
Should universal screening be part of an educational program? Should recipients of infected blood be notified?
Should contacts of infected persons be traced and notified?
How should contact tracing and notification be done? Is
voluntary testing advisable? If so, how should it be encouraged? What are the implications of mandatory screening or voluntary testing programs for people who test
positive? What should be done in response to positive
tests? These are vexing questions that raise complex and
profound issues of public policy and ethics.[11] The difficulties foreseen in responding to these concerns ought not,
however, be used as an excuse to ignore the public health
crisis that prompts them.

Preventing or slowing the AIDS epidemic through education must be a high priority. However, this objective

ought to be a companion to two other objectives: effective therapies for complications of HIV infection, and a cure for HIV infection. Many of the acute illnesses associated with AIDS are treatable by conventional therapies. These treatments frequently restore patients to a relative state of health that provides an acceptable quality of life. Unfortunately, some complications of HIV infection, like cryptosporidiosis and cryptococcal meningitis, either are not treatable or the treatments are less effective. These therapeutic responses to acute and chronic illnesses may cure or lessen the effects of a particular secondary disease, but they do not address the underlying immune defect that permits these illnesses to develop. Clearly, the primary objective of research is eradication of HIV and its destructive effect on the immune system and the central nervous system, without becoming inattentive to treating complications.

The experience of scientists and physicians since 1981 suggests that finding a cure is a formidable task. There is no doubt that the basic science and therapeutics of viral diseases are improving. Treatments for herpes, papilloma virus (wart virus), and cytomegalovirus are reducing or preventing the acute signs of infection, if not providing a cure. This experience with less lethal viruses is proving valuable in the fight against HIV. But HIV is a virus hard to combat because it infects not only blood cells but also brain cells and probably any number of other types of cells. Thus, ridding the body of HIV may be an unattainable objective, because to destroy the virus in cells may require destroying brain cells that cannot be replaced. Suppressing viral replication and preventing the infection of new cells may be the most practical approach, given the action of the virus in the body. Antiviral drugs must, as a consequence, cross the blood–brain barrier, be safe for long-term use, and be administered orally, so patients are not tied to intravenous modes of treatment, adversely affecting quality of life and straining the health care system. Finally, effective therapy should be low-cost, since there is an urgent need for therapy in poor countries.

Efforts to identify, develop, and test drugs that safely inhibit virus replication thus far have produced limited positive results. Many scientists and physicians believe that a two-pronged attack will be required: an antiviral drug and an immune stimulatory drug. The first offensive, an antiviral drug, would stop the destructive effect of HIV. The second offensive, an immune stimulator, would rebuild or stimulate the immune system. It is too early to determine which offensive will produce positive results first, or if a single agent is capable of attaining both ends. Until a cure of whatever description is found, physicians caring for AIDS, ARC, and LAS patients will only be able to respond to acute and chronic complications of HIV infection with the most effective therapies presently available.

For the population not infected by HIV, a protective vaccine is urgently needed in order to abort a rapidly developing epidemic. There are several feasible approaches to the development of a retroviral vaccine. Which of these approaches, if any, will be perfected is impossible to predict now. It is clear, however, that once a vaccine is developed, demonstrating its efficacy will require years of observation. Initial clinical trials of AIDS vaccines should begin in 1987. Whatever the outcome of these or subsequent trials, vaccination is not a solution to the present global crisis of AIDS and HIV-related diseases.

HIV and its clinical manifestations present an awesome and complex challenge to scientists and physicians. Intensive efforts are under way within the scientific community to develop a protective vaccine and to overcome the barriers to a cure for HIV infection. While these goals are being pursued, the pain, suffering, and death produced by HIV cannot be ignored. A compassionate response to everyone directly or indirectly experiencing the destructive effects of HIV is indicated. Such a response to people tragically touched by this insidious virus is an obligation, not an option, for the people of God.

3

Illness
in Christian
Perspective

The question of how to account for the existence of
illness, suffering, and tragedy as integral parts of daily life
has preoccupied the human psyche throughout history. In
particular, the Christian church has struggled with the
relationship of illness to faith. The Gospels provide little
insight regarding the role of illness and suffering in creation. Issues of how to justify the ways of God seem to have
been unimportant to Jesus, who clearly gave priority to
the urgency of proclaiming the gospel. We seemingly cannot forgo our human preoccupation with attempts to explain illness and suffering, but apparently Jesus did not
join these discussions. He was too busy going about healing the sick, casting out demons, and, in so doing, manifesting God's compassion and love toward the afflicted.
The church attempts to keep a balance between these two
functions, engaging in acts of compassion and support to
people in need and reflecting theologically on the relationship of this ministry to the church's confession and mission. If the New Testament is a guide, ministry must
remain in the forefront of the church's activity. But theology as critical reflection on the work of ministry is not a
secondary function. Rather, each function informs and
corrects the other; each fulfills a servant role, so that the
church's work may be done.[1]

It is important to pursue this interrelationship with respect to the AIDS epidemic. The dimensions of this crisis, the needs of people with AIDS, and societal reactions to people with AIDS demand a response from the church. We must discover the appropriate form such a response must take, as to both the nature of compassionate ministry and the theological imperatives by which care and concern are shaped and corrected. In the course of exploring these issues, we will discover that the scriptures do not offer simple answers to questions related to the existence of illness and suffering. Rather, they call the people of God to serve their neighbors. At this moment, that includes people with AIDS.

New Testament Perceptions of Suffering

The New Testament recognizes suffering as a part of daily living that must be accepted and endured with fortitude. The troubles to be borne in this earthly existence are of little consequence compared to the life that is "hidden with Christ in God" (Col. 3:3). The New Testament, however, addresses sufferings at three levels. First, some afflictions clearly were the consequences of imprisonment and persecution because of the believer's witness to faith in Jesus Christ as Lord. Thus was Stephen stoned to death. Second, suffering may be the result of oppression by one person or group of another person or group. The most frequently cited biblical example is the oppression of the weak and helpless by the wealthy and powerful. Third, pain and suffering may be due to disease or physical or mental disability.

Suffering "For Christ's Sake"

Peter refers to suffering "for Christ's sake," for example, when he warns his readers that they may suffer "trials of many kinds." These trials come so that their faith "may prove itself worthy of all praise, glory, and honour when Jesus Christ is revealed" (1 Peter 1:6–7). Paul expresses the same thought frequently. Writing to the Corinthians, he offers the example of his faithful witness:

> As God's servants, we try to recommend ourselves in all circumstances by our steadfast endurance: in distress, hardships, and dire straits; flogged, imprisoned, mobbed; overworked, sleepless, starving. . . . Dying we still live on; disciplined by suffering, we are not done to death; in our sorrows we have always cause for joy; poor ourselves, we bring wealth to many; penniless, we own the world."
>
> (2 Corinthians 6:4–5, 9–10)

One of the richest sources of this image is in the eleventh chapter of the same letter:

> Five times the Jews have given me the thirty-nine strokes; three times I have been beaten with rods; once I was stoned; three times I have been shipwrecked, and for twenty-four hours I was adrift on the open sea. I have been constantly on the road; I have met dangers from my fellow-countrymen, dangers from foreigners, dangers in towns, dangers in the country, dangers at sea, dangers from false friends.
>
> (2 Corinthians 11:23–26; see also, for example, Romans 8:19; 13–19; 1 Corinthians 4:9–13; 2 Corinthians 1:8–11; 4:8–12, 16–18)

These "trials of many kinds" were anticipated in phrases attributed to Jesus in the Beatitudes: "How blest you are, when you suffer insults and persecution and every kind of calumny for my sake. Accept it with gladness and exultation, for you have a rich reward in heaven; in the same way they persecuted the prophets before you" (Matt. 5:11–12). Suffering "for Christ's sake" on the part of his followers is thus incorporated into the suffering for the sake of righteousness that characterizes both Old and New Testaments. In the Old Testament, it is linked to the concept of the Suffering Servant. In the New Testament, Peter recognizes that such human suffering participates in the suffering of Christ:

> My dear friends, do not be bewildered by the fiery ordeal that is upon you, as though it were something extraordi-

nary. It gives you a share in Christ's sufferings, and that
is cause for joy; and when his glory is revealed, your joy
will be triumphant. . . . If anyone suffers as a Christian, he
should feel it no disgrace, but confess that name to the
honour of God.

(1 Peter 4:12–13, 16)

Such passages often seem to be advanced in support of the
claim that when suffering in the form of physical illness
is experienced, it ought to be accepted and endured as an
ordeal in the sense intended by Peter: that is, a trial sent
to test the believer's faith. A clear distinction, however,
should be made as to the source of the suffering before
physical hardship and illness are so linked, as will be
noted.

Suffering as the Result of Oppression

The Gospels note a second source of suffering against
which Jesus cried out in protest, and which is to be opposed at every point: suffering that results from human
injustice and oppression of the poor. Luke begins his record of Jesus' ministry with the account of the visit to
Nazareth. The words from Isaiah 61 are applied to the
ministry of Jesus: "[The Lord] has sent me to announce
good news to the poor" (Luke 4:18). The announcement
is clearly intended to address the concerns that so roused
the prophets: the need to proclaim liberation to broken
victims and release to the captives. It is usual to link with
these phrases the complementary passages from Isaiah.
Thus, the Gospel calls for the loosing of the fetters of
injustice, untying the knots of the yoke, snapping every
yoke, and setting free those who have been crushed. To the
cry for compassion toward the crushed is added the call
to proclaim recovery of sight to the blind and to clothe the
naked, provide hospitality to the homeless poor, feed the
hungry, and satisfy the needs of the wretched (Isa.
58:6–10). In denouncing the religious authorities, Jesus
pointed to their greed: "Beware of the doctors of the law.
. . . These are the men who eat up the property of widows,

while they say long prayers for appearance' sake; and they will receive the severest sentence" (Luke 20:45–47).

Luke is not alone among the Evangelists in identifying Jesus as championing the cause of the poor and oppressed, but his gospel is noteworthy for this emphasis. With Matthew, Luke cites Jesus' reply to John's disciples, who sought confirmation that Jesus was really "the coming one." Jesus' ministries of healing and liberation were explicit signs of the reign of God—for those who had eyes of faith to see. The fact that, in the liberating actions of Jesus, John possessed all the evidence he needed to satisfy his uncertainty leads to only one conclusion: the power of God is present in Jesus. In its presence, evil—in the form of oppression of the innocent, injustice levied against those too weak to speak for themselves, or exclusion of the humble from the community's concern and care—is being overturned. The message is clear. Evil cannot continue to exist in the presence of God's love.

The hospitality of the kingdom is extended without hesitation to those whom society has oppressed or ignored: the poor, the crippled, the lame, and the blind (Luke 14:21), those whose homes are the city's streets and alleys (v. 21) or the roads and hedges of the countryside (vs. 23–24). Such gracious acts are extended to people who, because of their very weakness, even their failure to thrive, are unable to return the gift of hospitality. That they cannot is the best reason for inviting them. The inability of the poor to return the kindness is the measure of their need of it. The words and actions of Jesus are those of confrontation: the causes and consequences of poverty, injustice, and exclusion from the community are to be opposed. Not only will those who oppress the poor not inherit the kingdom; even those who fail to minister to the least of the Lord's brothers and sisters will go away to eternal punishment, "to the eternal fire that is ready for the devil and his angels" (Matt. 25:41). Jesus accused the Pharisees of having no care for justice and the love of God, and the lawyers of loading men with intolerable burdens (Luke 11:42, 46). The scene in the temple in which the

money-changers' tables were overthrown and the pigeons
freed from their cages expresses the same sense of outrage
at the afflictions imposed on the poor. For the robbery
being practiced involved not only the fraudulent activities
of the money-changers against worshipers, but the stealing
of this house from God. "Moreover, the thefts from men
were not limited to the Temple precincts, as Jeremiah
knew, but included the dog-eat-dog practices outside the
Temple by men who then took part in the worship (Jer.
7:8–15)."[2]

Jesus' work in the temple was a prophetic sign of God's
wrath, in accordance with God's desire to make God's
house a place of worship for all nations. God had prom-
ised to bring foreigners and gather the outcasts to rejoice
in the benefits of the temple (Isa. 56:6–8). "It was this
promise which Jesus fulfilled and which the priests repu-
diated, so that this episode becomes an epitome of the
Messiah's whole career."[3] As a result, Christians are not
urged to accept or tolerate such affliction with passive
resignation; they are bidden to lift the yoke of oppression
and to fill the role of champions of the downtrodden. The
followers of Jesus walk in his footsteps only if they are
filled with a like concern for the poor (we discuss this
theme more comprehensively in chapter 4).

Suffering Due to Disease or Disability

Just as injustice cannot exist in the presence of the
Lord's anointed, neither can sickness endure against
God's power. The citing of the Isaianic passages (Luke
4:18–19) signals Luke's emphasis on Jesus' ministry to the
poor and oppressed, included among whom, true to the
Old Testament passages, are the sick and disabled in body
and mind. This aspect of the discussion should be set in
the context of the attribution of causality for sickness and
affliction, and the perceived relationship between illness or
disability and ritual defilement, that has characterized
Judeo-Christian thought. Judaism struggled with the notion that sickness was a consequence of sin and therefore

a punishment. Acts of healing were acknowledged by proving to a priest that the symptoms of disease or disability had vanished, whereupon the priest declared that the defilement was lifted and the formerly disabled person was restored to the community and to the full benefits of the law. Ritual defilement resulted from any affliction, since it was axiomatic that the disease would not have occurred if the victim's relationship with God was not disordered.[4]

It is in this context that the ministry of Jesus to the sick should be set. Jesus was at pains to discard the ancient attribution of illness or disability as punishment for some act of disobedience of God's law: that is, as God's retribution for human sin. The tradition was long and deep. Sirach, or ben Sira, the author of Ecclesiasticus, declared in the second century B.C. that

From the beginning good things were created for the good,
and evils for sinners.
The chief necessities of human life
are water, fire, iron, and salt,
flour, honey, and milk,
the juice of the grape, oil, and clothing.
All these are good for the godfearing,
but turn to evil for sinners.

There are winds created to be agents of retribution,
with great whips to give play to their fury;
on the day of reckoning, they exert their force
and give full vent to the anger of their Maker.
Fire and hail, famine and *deadly disease,*
all these were created for retribution;
beasts of prey, scorpions and vipers,
and the avenging sword that destroys the wicked.
They delight in carrying out his orders,
always standing ready for his service on the earth;
and when their time comes, they never disobey.
(Ecclesiasticus 39:25–31; emphasis added)

Sirach clearly reflected a popularly held perception against which Jesus protested. John records the disciples' questioning of Jesus regarding a blind man: "Rabbi, who

sinned, this man or his parents? Why was he born blind?"
Jesus responded: "It is not that this man or his parents
sinned; he was born blind so that God's power might be
displayed in curing him" (John 9:2–3). Jesus rejected the
notion that God had deliberately disabled this man—and,
conceivably, others—on account of sin, or merely to provide an opportunity to demonstrate God's power. Indeed,
Mark presents Jesus as requiring the disciples to keep
silent concerning such acts lest they be regarded by the
populace as merely displays of power designed to coerce
a positive response to the gospel—and thus be misunder-
stood. Luke records that Jesus was challenged to explain
the sufferings of the innocent: for example, the Galileans
slaughtered by Pilate and the eighteen upon whom the
tower of Siloam fell (Luke 13:1–9). An easy solution
would be to say, echoing Job's friends, that the fate of the
Galileans overtook them in the providence of God, a just
punishment for some iniquity of which they were doubt-
less guilty. While it is precisely this theory that Jesus
rejects, he does not advance any alternative explanation at
this point.[5] The question of the problem of suffering is
unanswered, for Jesus treats the story, and another that he
raises, as parables. And the whole issue of the parables is
the urgency of the gospel. It is this urgency which is
offered as the basis for the Johannine statement: "While
daylight lasts we must carry on the work of him who sent
me; night comes, when no one can work. While I am in
the world I am the light of the world" (John 9:4–5).

The issue for Jesus is the primacy of the gospel. He had
come into Galilee "proclaiming the Gospel of God"
(Mark 1:14). What followed, whether teaching, confronting, ministering compassionately, or healing, was the
manifestation of the power of God at work: "If it is by the
finger of God that I drive out the devils, then be sure
the kingdom of God has already come upon you" (Luke
11:20). The healing acts were entailed by the message he
proclaimed. Nothing, including disease and devils, could
impede the progress of the kingdom's unveiling or withstand its power. Hence, the Markan "secret": the healing

acts would only be correctly perceived when people recognized them as outbreaks of the kingdom's presence. In any other context, they would appear as mere "signs and wonders," which Jesus refused the Pharisees.

When one turns to examine how Jesus acted when confronted by human distress arising from disease and disability, the evidence is overwhelming: Jesus responded at every opportunity to relieve such affliction. Healing was often performed in a manner indicative of confrontation with illness. The Gospels identify Jesus as engaged in two types of healing activity: the driving out of demons and the healing of the sick and physically disabled. The twelve disciples were sent out with instructions to heal the sick, raise the dead, cleanse lepers, and cast out devils (Matt. 10:8). In Capernaum, the crowds brought to him all who were ill or possessed by devils (Mark 1:3). To Pharisees who urged him to escape from Herod, he replied, "Go and tell that fox, 'Listen: today and tomorrow I shall be casting out devils and working cures' " (Luke 13:32). The separate identification of the two activities suggests two functions. In the case of demon possession, the confrontation with evil is emphasized, but such actions are viewed in the context of the struggle between the power of the evil one and the power of God. Edward Schillebeeckx notes, "As Jesus pursues his ministry and manifests himself, this in itself is regarded by the evil powers as an act of aggression (Mk. 1:23–24 and parallels; 5:7ff. and parallels; 9:20–25). Against the evil and hurtful results produced by these powers Jesus sets only good actions, deeds of beneficence."[6]

The exorcisms are presented to show that God's eschatological kingdom is now present. Illness in general, however, was a sign of disorder in God's creation that ends with physical death. While sickness and death are customarily assumed to be evidence of the activity of evil, the healing of the sick is set in the context of the announcement of the kingdom and of Jesus' compassion for those who, because of their illness, are unable to live life to its fullest. Again and again, he is represented as reaching out to people at their points of need. Acts 10:38 states that witnesses can bear testimony to all that he did in the Jewish countryside and in Jerusalem: he went about doing good and healing all who were oppressed by the devil, "actively showing pity for the sick and those who by the standards of that time were held to be possessed by 'the demon' or by 'demons,' 'the prisoners' whom the eschatological prophet was to set free (Isa. 61:1–2)."[7] The commitment of Jesus on behalf of people in distress became the basis for the early church's emphasis on the preaching of the "glad tidings of Jesus Christ" (Mark 1:1). The Gospels report that the response of Jesus to those whose lives were disordered was one of tenderness and compassion. Nothing aroused his anger more spontaneously than unfeeling and uncaring legalists who saw not the distress of a person crippled in mind or body but an opportunity to moralize on the basis of some fine point of the Torah (Mark 3:1–6; see also Matt. 23:23: "You pay tithes of mint and dill and cummin; but you have overlooked the weightier demands of the Law, justice, mercy, and good faith. . . . Blind guides! You strain off a midge, yet gulp down a camel!").

The intensity of Jesus' response to human suffering is illustrated in the story of the healing of a man with a crippled hand (Mark 3:1–6). The healing is necessary on the Sabbath, since in Hebrew thought not to heal the man would leave him nearer to death—for sickness is proximity to death.[8] That is, the struggle against sickness is a struggle to save the sufferer from the power of death and the threat it poses. Since sickness opposes the Creator God's saving power, it must be righted and the creation restored. Jesus is the Redeemer in whom the mercy of God is present. What is new in his ministry is that the beneficiaries of God's mercy are not the religious authorities and legal scholars but those considered outsiders: the poor, the disabled, the sick, and the bereaved. Jesus made himself accessible to those who needed him, ignoring conventional limitations and thus according proper recognition to those who were cast out of society for whatever reason. Consistently, he met people at their particular points of need and addressed those needs. Jesus is presented as a combatant, constantly opposing with his power those forces that kept people in subjugation. Whatever held people back from experiencing the fullness of the gospel must be confronted and its power to do so destroyed. Thus, the sick were healed, the disabled returned to full activity, and the oppressed freed.

When Jesus welcomed the sick and disabled with open arms, he presented a potent model to his followers. The manner in which churches and their members respond to people with AIDS is an indication of the degree of seriousness with which they follow the example of Jesus. A response of love and compassion—an open-arms response— is demanded of God's people. It is a mandate expressly given by Jesus, as, for example, in the parable of the Judgment (Matt. 25:31–46). Further, such a response is a sign of God's gracious love, not only to people with AIDS and to their loved ones but to the wider community. It announces for all to see and hear that the kingdom is being realized, that it is taking shape in the world. If AIDS, in fact, means that the sick person has fallen into death's realm of power, loving acceptance of people with AIDS announces that God's saving power takes the field against death's destructive power.

During a recent hospitalization, a young man who knew that his struggle with numerous infections occasioned by AIDS was reaching its inevitable end drew comfort from the knowledge that his membership in a local church had led to the development of a support group for AIDS patients in the congregation. During the final days of his struggle he was visited by members of the group. His family gathered to support him. He was distressed that his family, in particular, would remember him racked with pain and broken by disease. With a supreme effort, he spent some time with each family member, leaving each with the message of how important was their support and love and how strong his love was for them. The ministry of the religious community was one of the undergirding forces in the hospital room, both for the patient and for his family. It symbolized God's gracious and reconciling love. Such compassion is a first call upon God's people in the crisis created by the AIDS epidemic.

The "Problem of Suffering"

In marked contrast to the fact that Jesus was concerned to show compassion to the afflicted rather than to establish the causes of disease and disability, Western scholars have tended to be preoccupied with the latter concern, connecting their response to issues of morality. The church's response to sickness and disability has been influenced by both emphases, which have existed side by side in Western culture. The ministry of compassion, so integral to the ministry of Jesus, is manifested, for example, in the establishment of an infirmary in Rome as early as the late fourth century, a logical development of Christian charity. The commandment to love the neighbor (Matt. 19:19; 22:39; Mark 12:31–33) was not simply a piece of advice, it was a categorical imperative. Love for the neighbor can be manifested in a variety of ways, but spiritual concern must never take precedence over immediate material or physical help for those in need, as the Letter of James bluntly states: "Religion that is pure and undefiled before God and the Father is this: to visit orphans and widows in their affliction" (1:27, RSV).

The visitation, care, and comfort of the afflicted became an obligation incumbent upon all Christians and was repeatedly stressed in early Christian literature. This duty to attend the sick and the poor conferred on them a preferential position that has lasted until now. The example of Christ was followed in the mid-third century when, during an outbreak of plague, Christians ministered to plague victims. In a letter by Dionysius written in A.D. 263, he describes how "our brethren were unsparing in their exceeding love and brotherly kindness. They held fast to each other and visited the sick fearlessly and ministered to them continually, serving them in Christ. . . . And many who cared for the sick and gave strength to others died themselves . . . so that this form of death, through the great piety and strong faith it exhibited, seemed to lack nothing of martyrdom."[9] The commitment to the outcast sick is evident in the nineteenth century exemplified by Fr. Damien on the island of Molokai, and into the twentieth century, with Mother Teresa and countless nameless people for whom the needs of the sick and dying become a call to ministry.

Yet this often sacrificial gesture of compassionate response has been accompanied by efforts to explain the existence of pain and suffering in terms of retribution. For example, Calvin identified two purposes served by suffering caused by such events as pestilence, disease, poverty, or any other suffering in body or mind. First, suffering is punishment for high crimes and misdemeanors against God, a punishment justly deserved. Calvin prayed that God's chastisements—the affliction of disease or poverty, for example—would be effective for the reformation of the sufferer's life. In this sense, suffering has an expiatory force which imparts the assurance to the believer that guilt is thereby atoned, reflecting the Talmudic statement that the one who has suffered in this life is thereby assured of rewards in the life to come. Second, suffering is perceived to have an educational purpose. Calvin directed ordained pastors who visit those afflicted by disease or "other evils" to

> console them by the word of the Lord, showing them that all which they suffer and endure comes from the hand of God, and from his good providence, who sends nothing to believers except for their good and salvation. . . . Moreover, if he sees the sickness to be dangerous, he will give them consolation, which reaches farther, according as he sees them touched by their affliction; that is to say, if he sees them overwhelmed by the fear of death, he will show them that it is no cause for dismay to believers, who having Jesus Christ for their guide and protector, will, by their afflic-

tion, be conducted to the life on which he has entered. By similar considerations he will remove the fear and terror which they may have of the judgment of God.[10]

This manner of presenting poverty and disease—and, in fact, misfortune generally—has endured into modern Western usage and remains a powerful influence on contemporary attitudes to disease and disability. During a morning TV news presentation late in 1986, the parents of a promising college athlete who had died during 1986 were interviewed. Asked what meaning they attached to their son's death, his mother responded that God had made their son an example to other youth "so that millions might live." The same attribution of suffering is evident in the tracts left in hospital waiting areas or placed on bedside tables that carry such messages as: *Sickness is an opportunity to mature inwardly; The Lord does not place burdens upon us that are more than we can bear; Affliction is God's test of our faith; we must pray for strength.*

It seems that either the experience of personal affliction or the awareness of suffering in another person inevitably drives humanity back to the question asked poignantly by the psalmists: Why do righteous people suffer? Attempts to answer that question seem endless. The Hebraic perception of God, which attributed all phenomena to a divine purpose, was carried over into early Christendom and remains a pervasive influence in much "folk religion." As the Renaissance paved the way ultimately for the enhancement of the sciences, however, larger and larger areas of human life were explained on the basis of a growing body of scientific data. Included in this explosion of knowledge was the matter of illness. A small group of British scientists was convened in the late 1950s to review the relationship between religion and science. The group recalled that in the Middle Ages people crowded into churches to seek deliverance from plagues, whereas twentieth-century societies dig drains and educate the public concerning matters of hygiene. Whereas primitive societies prayed for rain and abundant harvests, we invest resources in water conservation and teach third world countries the benefits of fertilizers and crop rotation. When humans were forced to account for phenomena they could not understand, the tendency was to fall back upon the age-old measure of attributing causality to some unfathomed divine purpose. The problem arose, however, that as rational explanations emerged to account for more and more areas of human experience, the extent of experience ascribed to a purposive God began to shrink. Now that science can explain in intricate detail the manner in which viruses enter and affect the human body, and how the body's immune system defends itself against such attacks, it is tempting to divide human experience into two (or more) parts, granting science control over one while retaining the control of religion over the other. This is a mistake. To assert that some sort of hedge can be planted in the country of the mind to mark the boundary where a transfer of authority takes place is a twofold error. First, it presupposes an intolerable dichotomy of existence. Second, it invites "science" to discover new things and thence gradually take possession of that which "religion" once held.[11] Soon, God becomes no longer necessary because the gap between the explained and the unexplained is closed. If this image is applied to the science of medicine, any attempt to remove disease from the arena of medicine to that of religion assumes the same dichotomization, an untenable position. God does not reserve certain areas of life in which to dabble. In particular, AIDS was not "sent" on some divine intention to communicate a message; for example, to remind humans that God retains some areas in which to manifest initiative.

There is a second and more disturbing objection to the notion that the answer to suffering is to be found in some divine purpose. Dorothee Soelle put the issue forcefully when she objected to what she termed "theological sadism." For her, "Christian masochism," had "so many features that merit criticism: the low value it places on human strength; its veneration of one who is neither good nor logical but only extremely powerful; its viewing of suffering exclusively from the perspective of endurance; and its consequent lack of sensitivity for the suffering of others." But what bothered Soelle was not the well-meaning attempts of onlookers to comfort a disabled person; such attempts may be genuine efforts to speak in comfort and compassion. Her greatest discomfort and anger arose because "the picture changes as soon as theologians, in a kind of overly rigorous application of the masochistic approach, sketch in as a companion piece a sadistic God." Her concern was that such a God who causes affliction and suffering is presented as one who demands the impossible and then tortures people.[12]

As this chapter was being written, a father sat for three weeks at the bedside of his dying twenty-eight-year-old son. He dealt with his grief out of images derived from the Middle Ages. He stated simply that what was happening was God's will, which he had no alternative but to accept. When the chaplain asked how he would feel if he were to discover that his son's imminent death was not "willed" by God but that instead God "grieved" over the death of one of God's children, he dismissed the image without consideration. The chaplain did not return to the theological issue; at that moment such a discussion was not appropriate. The father's conviction that his son's death was at God's behest was his only source of comfort. It might have been easier to accept his perception if his consolation had been deep and genuine. But it was as if he were engaged in a never-ending struggle to hold back the waters of bitterness behind a narrow dike, with his finger plunged into a fissure through which the waters seeped, constantly threatening to become a surge that would overwhelm him. Similarly, a hospital chaplain recounted a ten-year-old patient's struggle to come to terms with his diagnosis of AIDS. Who knows the source of the child's images? Had some well-meaning relative, friend, or pastor sought to comfort him by suggesting gently that God had "chosen" him? He sat up in bed and cried out, "Why did God choose me? I did not want to be chosen!"

These images of God are derived from perceptions of

God's transcendence that leave little room for immanence such as manifested in the life of Jesus of Nazareth, who sat beside a woman alienated from her community, or who crouched in a dusty village street alongside another threatened woman. These biblical pictures contrast sharply with the image of a transcendent God, far removed from human concerns except to use them as teaching opportunities. It is right to criticize radically all attempts to reconcile God with misery or, worse, to represent God as sanctioning misery. Such a God, who uses affliction merely or primarily to reprove, correct, or educate, cannot be separated from the accusation of injustice. If God "comes to a sufferer only with pedagogical intent,"[13] then God seems deaf to the anguished protest of a ten-year-old child or any other person with AIDS, on whose behalf all must cry out for justice and compassion.

To attribute suffering to an all-powerful God who uses such power to inflict pain and misery upon humanity flies in the face of the incarnation of God's love in Jesus Christ. Such love is expressed in an active goodwill toward people, moved by a genuine sensitivity to their deepest needs. This type of love includes, but is not limited to, compassionate sympathy. Sympathy indeed has received a bad press, with the contemporary emphasis by social scientists on terms such as "empathy." Sympathy involves being present with a person—weeping with the sad, rejoicing when there is cause for celebration. It is comforting for one who is sick to know that he or she is not alone and that others care. "Empathy," on the other hand, is a construct that more fully expresses a human attempt to speak of God's love. The term involves a relationship between the helper and the afflicted person in which the helper knows, or can imagine, the depth of the pain and struggle the other is experiencing. It is a relationship that opens the possibility of change or, if that is not possible, assures the struggler that the helping person has the ability to enter into the feeling of helplessness or even despair and know what it means. If these images may be applied validly to God's love, they suggest that God is in touch with our pain, that God "feels" our anguish and is affected by it. This conception is in stark contrast to the Greek notion of divine impassibility that has permeated traditional theism, a notion that sharply restricts the biblical perception of divine love that is responsive to human suffering. The idea that God's knowledge of the world is complete and unchanging implies that God has determined every aspect of the world, down to the last detail. Nothing can happen that is not immutably known. There is little provision for creaturely freedom in such a fixed system. Process theology, on the other hand, sees God's creative activity as based upon responsiveness to the world. Since the very meaning of actuality involves internal relatedness, God as an actuality is essentially related to the world. Since actuality as such is partially self-creative, future events are not determined. Even perfect knowledge, process theologians argue, cannot know the future. Thus, God does not wholly control the world. God's power, even creative power, is persuasive, not coercive.[14]

Process thought has three immediate consequences for this inquiry. First, it provides a theological basis for the assertion that God does not select specific diseases to punish certain human behaviors. If God's power is persuasive, not controlling, finite actualities can fail to conform to the divine aims for them. Deviations from divine aims may give rise to evil. Since deviation is possible, though not necessary, evil is not necessary. It is the *possibility* of deviation that is necessary, and that makes the *possibility* of evil necessary. The risk in all this for humanity is that a new actuality may develop which introduces a novel element into creation. It may add to the variety of existence, and so to the value that can be enjoyed. But the new reality may be a strain of virus which leads not to enjoyment but to discord.[15] Human immunodeficiency virus (HIV) surely falls into this category. If the intention had been to exclude the possibility of all discord, God would simply have abstained from creating a world altogether, and so have guaranteed the absence of all suffering. Risk is part of the created order, a price paid for freedom,

God's trump card. Thus, God does not "send" AIDS for some retributive purpose (such a thought flies in the face of the New Testament witness to a loving God). Rather, God "risked" creating a world in which HIV could develop.

The second consequence of process thought centers around the question of persuasiveness vs. control. It is on just this issue that conservative Christians oppose radically any stance to the left of their own positions. "Fundamentalist" and "liberal" Christians may fight over matters of ecclesiology and biblical and historical theology, but what is at stake is the political issue of management styles and measures of control and freedom. This battle has certainly invaded areas of ethics and theology in accounting for human suffering, but it also plays a key role in the form that pastoral care takes—for example, in shaping attitudes toward people with AIDS. Care and compassion can be offered to people in need without attempting to coerce them into adopting the caregiver's religious commitments. It is appropriate for ministries to reflect religious and moral values; it is not appropriate, however, to expect the other person to adopt those values as the *condition* for the relationship and the care.[16]

Both the Hebrew scriptures and the New Testament characterize God as choosing to deal freely with humanity. God offers humanity choices. The question then is whether the choices made are trivially or morally evil or are genuine attempts at responsible living. This matter of choice is always unambiguous. It is the choice expressed by Joshua to the Israelities: "Hold the Lord in awe then, and worship him in loyalty and truth. Banish the gods whom your fathers worshipped beside the Euphrates and in Egypt, and worship the LORD. But if it does not please you to worship the LORD, choose here and now whom you will worship. . . . I and my family, we will serve the LORD" (Josh. 24:14–15). The choice is presented as sharply by Jesus to the rich young ruler: "Jesus said to him, 'If you wish to go the whole way, go, sell your possessions, and give to the poor . . . and come, follow me' " (Matt. 19:21).

The fact of freedom places the responsibility for decision and choice on the only one who can assume such responsibility, the person who must decide. The attempt to control the choices of others is a constant temptation for caregivers. One of the temptations is to reject a person who has made a decision with which one disagrees or, more pointedly, which is offensive to one's own moral judgment. It is also tempting to use the power implicit in the role of the caregiver to overwhelm the person who needs help and to make help contingent upon the adoption of an "acceptable" lifestyle.[17]

This raises the third consequence of process thought for this inquiry. It is logical to argue that if God's relationship with humanity is persuasive, that characteristic should be the model for our own interpersonal relationships. It should apply particularly to the role of caregiver. If persuasion, rather than control, is the divine mode of relation, this manner of doing things is expected of believers. These images of relationship—offer, freedom, and persuasion—are true to the gospel. The object of preaching the gospel is "full life" (John 10:10). That invitation is offered, but in large measure it is up to each of us how that full life will be appropriated. God's creative purpose for humanity is loving because God is always a completely *gracious* God. God's aim for people is existence that they experience as intrinsically good. But God is not in complete control. We are in part responsible for who we are and what we shall become. We are certainly responsible for the choices we make and for their consequences. The freedom God offers humanity is therefore risky, but it is a necessary risk if there is to be the chance for greatness. Thus the question as to whether God is indictable for evil reduces to the question of whether the positive values enjoyed by the higher forms of life and experience are worth the risk of the negative values; namely, the sufferings. Should humans, therefore, risk possible suffering in order to have at least the possibility of intense enjoyment? Process theologians Cobb and Griffin respond affirmatively, explaining that the divine reality is an Adventurer who not only enjoys humanity's experience of the pitch of enjoyment but who also experiences sufferings.[18] God knows what it is like to taste the bitter waters of our valleys of Marah (Ex. 15:23).

The desert plains across which lie our paths, as we press forward looking for Canaan, that land flowing with milk and honey, are broken by more than one valley of Marah. The ancient pilgrimage of the children of Israel remains a prototype for all. AIDS is but the latest tragedy to evoke from humanity the age-old question, "Why, Lord? Why me?"

It has been suggested that from the most primitive of ancient cultures to the more highly developed religious forms, humanity has always struggled with the tragedy of affliction, resolving the paradox of life pockmarked by suffering by attributing disease and disability to the gods' anger at human failure and sin. Primitive Hebrew thought incorporated this concept, and much of contemporary Christian "folk religion" reflects it. Yet the biblical response is one of affirmation. It does not answer the question, "Why me?" other than to remind us, through metaphor, that we are called to be children of our Father in heaven, who makes the sun rise on good and bad alike and sends the rain on the honest and dishonest (Matt. 5:45). We are assured that God makes those whom society denigrates God's people. It is salutary to remember that the first epistle of Peter was addressed to just such people: domestics, street sweepers, laborers, and Gentiles. The writer's joy is in seeing people who once were "no people" becoming "God's people." Those who had not previously received mercy were now recipients of God's mercy. Nobodies were receiving the dignity and the joy of being God's children. Is there any comfort for a patient in the theological notion that his or her God, who has rejoiced in human achievements and enjoyments, now shares in the pain and physical discomfort of his or her dying?

There is no formula for erasing the pain and anguish of people with AIDS and of their loved ones. Moreover, as

sick and disabled people constantly remind those who just
stand around, one who has not experienced catastrophic
crisis cannot know the feelings it evokes in the sufferer.
But in the face of such pain, the witness of scripture is
plainly and simply stated: God is a God of unfathomable
love who tends people like a shepherd tends the flock. The
human analogy is of a loving parent who loves to the
uttermost. This affirmation moves Paul to reassure his
readers that nothing can separate people from the love of
God revealed in the Christ. Not persecution, hunger,
nakedness, peril, or sword; not illness, disability, or AIDS.
But our thoughts are not God's thoughts; neither are our
ways God's ways. We do not rise to Paul's level of maturity but continue to judge from our human point of view.
We cannot say, with the apostle, that "worldly standards
have ceased to count in our estimate of any man" (2 Cor.
5:16). So we continue to place people in categories, creating new groups of "the poor" from whom, because they
do not fit our stereotypes, we distance ourselves.

4

God
and the Poor

Illness and disability are seen in scripture as opportunities for God's people to provide compassionate care and protection. The record of the church's ministries of visitation, health care, and asylum demonstrates the seriousness with which the biblical examples and admonitions have been taken. These ministries are extensions of Jesus' ministry and represent creative responses to the command to love one's neighbor.

Sick and disabled persons are only two instances within a broader category of persons toward whom the people of God are to be benevolently disposed—the poor. "The poor" is a theological metaphor representing that collection of persons in biblical society who were vulnerable to exploitation or were afforded less than an equal place because of their condition or situation in life. The poor were people who were without the necessary human or material resources to protect their welfare or to secure their place in society.

The Poor in Jewish Scripture

Within the speeches of Moses reported in Deuteronomy, Israel is told that living in covenant with God requires nothing less than total loyalty and obedience to the

Holy One. Israel is to have an attitude of reverence toward God, to live according to God's instructions, to love God, and to serve God without reservation. Moses describes this God who merits and commands such service as one who "secures justice for widows and orphans, and loves the alien who lives among you, giving him food and clothing" (Deut. 10:18). Orphans, widows, and aliens in Jewish culture were potential victims of social and legal abuse. Their ally and defender is God; and Israel, in imitation of God, is to stand as God does in relation to these people.

Other biblical passages also identify the orphan, the impoverished, and the stranger as subject to God's special protection (e.g., Ex. 22:21–27; Lev. 19:33–34). "Weak" and "poor" were used by the prophets as terms for these people and others who could not maintain their own support or status in society and who, as a consequence, were particularly vulnerable to exploitation or to having their rights violated. They are those whom society tends to treat unjustly and to whom few offer comfort, defense, or care. They are people who tend to be forgotten and whose claims are ignored by those with power and prestige. They are people who are marginalized by social structures, practices, and dominant values. The witness of scripture, however, is that God is their ally (Isa. 3:15), advocate (Ex. 22:21–24), and protector (Isa. 25:4; 41:17). God's concern for the poor is so great, according to Isaiah, that the manner in which they are protected is the divine, functional measure of whether or not a society is just (Isa. 3:14–15).

The situation of the poor was seen as the result of social factors rather than as a consequence of personal failings. They were people with little power, victims of fate in need of compassion, or victims of injustice in need of justice (Isa. 10:2). The great expression of God's will for the oppressed was the liberation of Israel from slavery in Egypt. God heard the cry of the oppressed covenant people and restored them to a position of power and freedom (Ex. 2:23–24). This event became the prototype and standard by which Israel's response to oppression and injustice was to be measured. In addition, the memory of Israel's enslavement was frequently invoked by God's messengers as a motivation not to abuse the rights of the socially and legally weak. The refrain "for you were strangers in the land of Egypt" (e.g., Ex. 22:21; 23:9, RSV) beckoned the people to identify with the suffering of the weak and resist the temptation to neglect or exploit the vulnerable. The witness in Jewish scripture is that the needs of the poor and weak must be recognized and met. The prophets especially were sensitive to the legitimate needs of individuals and groups in society. Their pronouncements were calls to righteousness as much as they were pronouncements of judgment. Isaiah, speaking for God, entreats Judah: "Wash yourselves; make yourselves clean; remove the evil of your doings from before my eyes; cease to do evil, learn to do good; seek justice, correct oppression; defend the fatherless, plead for the widow" (Isa. 1:16–17, RSV). The prophet assumes that it is possible for people to change when the contrast between what they do and the way of righteousness is made known to them. According to the prophets, power was to be used to promote the welfare and rights of others. Nevertheless, the prophets surely were realistic. They must have known that no temporal society would be perfect. But their understanding of humanity and social relationships was perceptive enough to recognize that the character of any society reflects the character of the people who shape and control it. Thus the prophets' passion was for individuals and society to obey the will of God. In the words of Micah: "He has showed you, O man, what is good; and what does the Lord require of you but to do justice, and to love kindness, and to walk humbly with your God?" (Micah 6:8, RSV).

Central to the Bible's teachings regarding the poor is the conviction that they are subjects of divine concern and therefore worthy of just and merciful treatment. Though their positions in society were inferior, their needs and rights were to be given the same regard as the needs and rights of society's more privileged and secure members.

All persons, weak or strong, were equal under God and therefore were to be treated with equal respect (Ex. 21–23). The objective of the various commands regarding orphans (e.g., Ex. 22:22; Isa. 1:17), widows (Isa. 1:23; 10:2; Deut. 14:29), and strangers (Lev. 9:33–34; Ex. 22:21; 23:9)—that is, the poor—was to empower the vulnerable, to remind the strong of the equality of the weak before God, and to provide security for the poor. Since God was the source of all justice and righteousness, the rights and needs of everyone in the land, members and nonmembers of the covenant community alike, were to be respected.

By the time of the prophets, the interests of society as a whole were too easily identified with the interests of the ruling classes in maintaining their position and privilege. The interests of the poor tended to be ignored or minimized. As a consequence, the community, common purpose, and quality of common life that God willed tended to be obscured (Isa. 5:1–7; Hos. 1:9; Amos 5:23–24). God's anger toward Israel for these failures was not "the cold anger of a judge upholding law, but the passionate anger of a master whose goodness has been flouted, of a guardian whose helpless wards have been maltreated"[1] (Isa. 1:2–3; Hos. 11:1–4, 8–9). The prophets who denounced Israel's transgressions and called the nation to repentance were "social revolutionaries" because they were "religious conservatives" articulating the essential ethics and social creativity of historic Yahwism. Yahweh was in the struggle for social justice, and Israel, God's elect, was to participate in that struggle. God was the ally of the wronged and disadvantaged, and Israel, in loyalty and obedience to God, was to be their ally as well.

Together with this knowledge of God, Israel's concern for the poor was to be motivated by the memory of their experience in Egypt (e.g., Ex. 23:9; Deut. 15:11; 16:12). Fulfilling the duty of the strong to protect and care for the weak was not considered a burden; it was a privilege (Job 31:16–22). God did not look favorably upon indifference, abuse of the weak, or abuse of privilege. The people could not mask their corruption and failures with piety (Isa.

1:10–17). God could see through the pretense. The warning in Proverbs applied to all who ignored the cries of the poor and weak: "He who closes his ear to the cry of the poor will himself cry out and not be heard" (Prov. 21:13, RSV). God is a loving, empowering, liberating being who wills community and justice in human history, and the divine will is to be carried out by human beings, individually and corporately. Beyond all ethnic boundaries, God values justice and compassion for all.

The value of the poor to God and the importance of their place in the community are evidenced in and through the legislation and exhortations regarding their treatment. The poor were not to be maltreated and their needs were to be met. For example, a primary purpose of the law requiring a man to marry his brother's widow was to provide her with security (Deut. 25:5–10; cf. Lev. 22:13). The immigrant or resident alien was to be protected like the widows and orphans who were members of the covenant community (Ex. 22:21–22). Some grain and fruit was to be left unharvested, to be gleaned by the poor, fatherless, widow, stranger, or traveler (Lev. 19:9–10). A tenth of one's produce or income every three years was to be committed to the poor (Deut. 26:12). The specific provisions of these rules are less significant than the principle they express: the poor are valued and deserve compassion.

By being benevolent toward the poor, one honors God and is blessed by God (e.g., Prov. 14:21). But when the rulers or ordinary people fail to provide for and protect the weak, God is insulted (v. 31). God's parental anger is stirred and judgment falls on the offending authority or people (Deut. 27:19; Mal. 3:5). God's passion for the weak, vulnerable, powerless, and displaced is a recurring theme in Jewish scripture. The manner in which the strong and privileged are to meet their obligations toward the needy is variously expressed. A substantive, yet deceptively simple, compound truth emerges through these expressions of Israel's understanding of God and God's will for human relationships: God's love is not conditioned by social role or status, unless an individual is among the

poor. In that case, God's alliance with that person is paramount, because other individuals and society have failed
in their duties to act justly and compassionately toward
them.

Jesus and the Poor

God's concern for the outcasts and the poor depicted in
Jewish scripture is echoed in the New Testament, especially the Synoptic Gospels. The Evangelists demonstrate
that the poor are a primary concern of Jesus, both in his
teaching and in his ministry. Identifying with the prophetic tradition in Israel, Jesus recognized that people
whose situation excluded them from full participation in
the social, religious, and legal institutions should not be
considered beyond the scope of God's love and human
regard. His message and mission were explicit challenges
to the prevailing notions of who was acceptable to God
and for what reasons. He scandalized the official custodi-
ans of religion and morality by proclaiming an inclusive
message rather than an exclusive one. His behavior was a
living testimony of God's will to have fellowship with all.
The fact that Jesus' opponents reviled him, calling him a
glutton and drunkard, and criticized him for being a
friend of tax collectors and sinners is evidence that he
practiced what he preached (Matt. 11:19; Mark 2:16;
Luke 7:34). Jesus' opponents were unable or unwilling to
celebrate the redemptive, liberating, and inclusive activity
of God, powerfully symbolized in the table fellowship of
Jesus (Luke 14:15–24).

Jesus' concern for the needy reflects his radical sense of
an egalitarianism of the coming end of the age. His offer
to have fellowship with the outcast is an explicit repudia-
tion of temporal norms of worth and status (Mark 2:15–
17). It also is an expression of Jesus' belief that all people
are valued by God and that God's will for relationship
excludes no one. Greatness, according to Jesus, had little
to do with one's piety or conformity to the letter of the
law. Instead, true greatness is tied to one's ability to recog-

nize the worth and importance of people normally considered least important in society (Luke 9:46–48). In Jesus' day, for example, the least important included children, women, sinners, tax collectors, the impoverished, publicans, prostitutes, and the sick. The message and example of Jesus was that it is God's will and humanity's responsibility to find ways to enable these outcasts to participate fully in the ongoing life of the community (Luke 14:12–14). The means by which this goal is to be achieved, according to the example and teaching of Jesus, is through humility and service (Luke 14:7–11; 17:7–10; 22:24–27). Charity and care for persons, according to Jesus, are central to a life of discipleship.[2] Self-centeredness and self-righteousness are impediments to the sort of edifying, loving relationships that God wills for people.

In Jesus' time, "sinner" was a general category of persons notorious for violating the commandments of God. It also was a term for people engaged in despised occupations which were seen to lead to immorality or dishonesty, such as dice gamblers, usurers, tax collectors, and herdsmen (see Luke 18:11). Tax collectors, or publicans, especially were hated by the people. They were subtenants of wealthy toll farmers, who made the highest bid to collect the toll or tax from an area for a fixed period. They extracted the appropriate toll and an additional sum as profit (Luke 3:12–13), exploiting the public's ignorance of the toll scale for their own gain. As a consequence of their evil actions, publicans were denied civil rights and honorary offices, and were prohibited from testifying in trials. Repentance meant abandoning the profession and restoring what was unjustly taken, plus one fifth of the total. Given the scope and degree of their deception, repentance virtually was impossible. Their segregation from community life on moral grounds was practically irreversible.

Despite the moral condemnation and social ostracism directed toward publicans and others similarly situated, Jesus had fellowship with them, undeterred by their conduct or the societally mediated judgment of their actions. In addition to these despised and ostracized individuals, the company of Jesus was described by his opponents as the "little ones" (Mark 9:42), the "least" (Matt. 25:40, 45, RSV), or the "simple" (Matt. 11:25). These designations were applied to the religiously uneducated, the backward, the irreligious people in Palestinian society. Yet, as the gospels reveal, these people were among the followers of Jesus. People whose religious ignorance or moral misdeeds were barriers to salvation, according to the prevailing views of Jesus' time, were the predominant groups among Jesus' following. Jesus called them the poor (Luke 6:20), people who "labor and are heavy laden" (Matt. 11:28, RSV).[3]

The meaning Jesus gave to the poor is based on the use of the term in Luke 4:18 and its parallel in Matthew 11:5. The setting is the synagogue in Nazareth. Jesus read a composite of Isaiah 61:1–2 and 58:6: "The Spirit of the Lord is upon me, because he has anointed me to preach good news to the poor. He has sent me to proclaim release to the captives and recovering of sight to the blind, to set at liberty those who are oppressed, to proclaim the acceptable year of the Lord" (Luke 4:18–19, RSV). Luke conspicuously omits from the reading "to proclaim . . . the day of vengeance of our God" (Isa. 61:2, RSV). Afterward Jesus announces, "Today this scripture has been fulfilled in your hearing" (Luke 4:21, RSV). The eschatological, messianic mission that Isaiah foresaw, according to Jesus, was being inaugurated in his ministry. His was a mission of salvation and inclusion, not judgment and exclusion. Unlike the Baptist, who heralded the coming kingdom and pronounced judgments (Matt. 3:1–2), Jesus announced salvation for the poor. This whole incident in the synagogue at Nazareth prefigures the ministry of Jesus and the primitive church. It is the opening scene in an unfolding drama in Luke–Acts in which fellowship and salvation are extended to all persons, regardless of cultic, national, racial, moral, or social prejudices.

Jesus' opponents criticized his fellowship with the despised and outcast, asking the disciples: "Why does your teacher eat with tax collectors and sinners?" Jesus responded, "Those who are well have no need of a physician, but those who are sick. Go and learn what this means, 'I desire mercy, and not sacrifice.' For I came not to call the righteous, but sinners" (Matt. 9:11–13, RSV). Jesus' teaching and lifestyle were clear repudiations of the view that the letter of the law was more important than the spirit of the law. The revelation of God that was intended to facilitate redemption and fellowship was being distorted to become a barrier to the fulfillment of God's purposes. As a consequence, God's invitation through Jesus was received by people who recognized their needs, rather than by those who had needs but refused to recognize them. Neither John the Baptist nor Jesus demanded in principle that toll collectors, for example, must give up their profession as a condition for fellowship. Jesus met all outcasts as they were in the midst of their situation, and offered them fellowship.

The good news that Jesus brought to the poor was that they are invited to God's festive meal. Jesus dramatized the forgiveness he was offering in action, most impressively in his table fellowship with sinners. Jesus invited sinners into his house (Luke 15:2) and dined with them in festive meals (Mark 2:15–18). It was an honor to be invited to a meal. An invitation was an offer by the host of peace, trust, brotherhood, and forgiveness. Thus by table fellowship, by lodging with a toll collector (Luke 19:5), and by calling publicans to be his disciples (Mark 2:14), Jesus demonstrated that God had accepted the despised, the outcast, and the poor.

Given this background regarding Jesus' concern for the poor, the full meaning of the First Beatitude becomes clearer. The poor are blessed because the reign of God belongs to them alone (Luke 6:20). Salvation can be received only by people who recognize their need. Sinners, publicans, and prostitutes, according to the Gospels, will be acceptable to God, whereas the righteous who believe their place to be secure will discover that they have no place at all (e.g., Luke 18:14). In solidarity with the poor and outcast, Jesus takes upon himself their hurt from being declared outside the realm of concern. His declaration that God, too, stands in solidarity with the marginalized because of God's compassion and concern for justice was, as the Gospels reveal, intolerable to the power and status brokers concerned to preserve their privilege.

Jesus' unconditional offer to have fellowship with everyone, especially the poor, aroused the opposition of the religious establishment. Nevertheless, Jesus continued to violate official religious and social protocol in order to take the good news to people in need. Sexual, social, and cultic barriers were broken; risks were assumed in order to communicate God's inclusive message. Prejudice, regardless of its source or agency of mediation, did not inhibit the witness of God's agent. Some of Jesus' most dramatic acts of ministry—feeding, healing, casting out, forgiving— were directed toward people who had been abandoned or squeezed out according to the dominant values in society. In the language of liberation theology, Jesus made an option for the poor.

Opting for the poor means to opt for people, acting and living in a way that respects the inherent value of all to God, especially those who are not treated with respect according to prevailing social norms. Living in this manner may result in a radical change in lifestyle, approach to work, political concerns, or understanding of the faith community. Following the example of Jesus may entail a change in priorities; a higher priority for people and a suspicion of social norms that oppress and divide people (Matt. 19:16–22).

Opting for the poor also has a social component that subjects social structures or institutions to claims of justice and mutuality. People oppressed by social structures have their self-image and their lifestyle determined by the definitions, priorities, and interests of the powerful people and institutions within society. Equality, concern for others, and social change occur in such a situation when the oppressed assert their just claims for regard and when at least a few oppressors acknowledge the legitimacy of those claims. This is an implicit act of repentance by the former oppressors, who then are freed to progress from a dialogue between stronger and weaker to a solidarity of strong and weak in the struggle for total liberation. The biblical prototypes of widow, orphan, poor, hungry, thirsty, naked, sick, and stranger are symbols of otherness. The symbols and, moreover, the actual people they represent are a call to community and solidarity, a limitation to self-interest forged on the anvil of justice. Their claim to hospitality helps to shape moral consciousness. They expose selfishness and summon us to repentance. They call others to be moral and to enter into solidarity with them. The solidarity or community which results from the answered call is not due, according to this reasoning, solely to guilt. It occurs because the value of the stranger to humanity and to God is perceived and affirmed. It occurs because each stranger accepts responsibility for all other strangers.

Solidarity with and compassion for outcast and oppressed people—the poor—constitute an implicit criticism and explicit rejection of being content with the way things are rather than striving to conform things to the way God intends them to be. Solidarity and compassion, accordingly, are key features of prophetic ministry, which is an active ministry, embracing the pain and suffering of people, reminding people with power to lessen these burdens and that oppression in any form is an affront to God (Prov. 17:5). Thus, God's people are called to be prophets, to oppose the conditions that generate and perpetuate human deprivation, indignity, and oppression (Isa. 1:17; Amos 5:14–15). By so doing, God's people respond to God's love and compassion for all revealed in the humanitarian legislation of Israel, in the oracles of Israel's prophets, and in the person and ministry of Jesus.

The Poor in Our Midst

We have seen that the poor are described in scripture as widows, orphans, the fatherless, sojourners, strangers, the impoverished, afflicted, enslaved, oppressed, sick, thirsty, hungry, and naked, sinners, prostitutes, tax collectors, or publicans. Regardless of their specific social role, the poor were people who could be placed in one or more of the following categories: (1) a person without the resources necessary to maintain his or her support or status in society; (2) a person devalued and scorned according to the dominant values and norms; (3) a person whose rights and claims tended to be easily ignored, rendering him or her vulnerable to exploitation and abuse; or (4) a person whose inferior status was socially conferred, enforced, and alleged to reflect God's estimate of that person. It is not surprising, given these conditions and estimations, that the poor were people whose anguish was overlooked, whose cries for compassion and justice were ignored, and whose divinely conferred value and dignity were disregarded.

God's revelation made several counterclaims. (1) The poor are loved by God and deserve compassion. (2) God hears poor people's cries of distress and is their hope for deliverance. (3) God's people, in loyalty and obedience to God, are to recognize the needs of the poor and meet them. Despite these pronouncements and affirmations, the poor generally remained segregated and oppressed during the biblical era because of the dominance of cultic, national, racial, moral, and social barriers that tended to serve the interests of the privileged at the expense of the poor. The intensity of the opposition that Jesus encountered indicates how threatening a ministry to the poor can be to a society's sense of security and order.

Expanding the scope of our concern to include people who are different, disadvantaged, or unfortunate entails the risk that the encounter may prompt a questioning of our privileges and the values and structures that support them. Yet this examination and the changes that could ensue ought not deter God's people from seeking the poor. An encounter with them should result in an inclusive and loving response. There is no other option for the people of God if they are to be true to their identity and faithful to their calling. The biblical witness allows no exceptions and accepts no excuses. As long as there are people who are included among the poor according to the criteria just identified, God's people are required not only to welcome them as neighbors, and to extend hospitality to them, but to identify fully with them as members of God's family.

People with AIDS, almost without exception, satisfy one or more of the criteria for being included among the biblical category of the poor. Their physical and fiscal losses often make them almost totally dependent on others, unable to provide for themselves, and ineffective advocates of their interests. They are often feared and ostracized in society because of their disease. If the person is gay, bisexual, or an IV drug user, these labels are cited as an additional justification for relegating him or her to the edges of society. The rights of marginalized people are nonexistent, since such people tend to be unable, and few others seem willing, to assert and defend those rights. Finally, the label of gay, bisexual, drug user, or person with AIDS is a stigma reflecting society's condemnation. Moreover, AIDS is seen by some people to validate society's censure of those whose sexual identity or lifestyle is considered unacceptable. Clearly, people with AIDS are contemporary manifestations of the poor who, despite society's judgments to the contrary, are loved by God and deserve to be treated compassionately by God's people.

The AIDS poor, however, are not only those people diagnosed with AIDS. The category includes people diagnosed with AIDS-related complex and people infected with the AIDS virus. Both groups often are subject to the same disregard and disparaging treatment, which makes them functional equivalents to people with AIDS. In addition, family and friends of people in each of these classes become a component of the AIDS poor. Because of their association with people with AIDS, they tend to experience the isolation, stigma, and hopelessness so familiar to people with an AIDS-related diagnosis. The circle of the AIDS poor expands as more and more people worldwide become infected and become clinically ill as a consequence.

The challenge that the poor presented to the religious establishment during the first century confronts us today in people touched by AIDS. In both situations the people of God are called upon to affirm what the law, prophets, and Jesus proclaimed: God loves all humanity and desires to have fellowship with all humanity. Like Jesus, the church is to be involved in prophetic and servant ministries that express this truth by word and deed. The church is under scriptural warrant not to ignore or be indifferent to the suffering of any person or group, even if that person or group is judged unacceptable and unlovable by society.

AIDS is more than a challenge to the church. It sets before the church an opportunity to reflect on its identity and its mission. If the church fails to act compassionately, neglects the needs that cluster around people with AIDS, fails to express itself redemptively, and abandons people who have almost no one to cry out on their behalf for mercy and justice, then the church will abdicate its responsibility and fail in its witness.

5
AIDS Ministries

As churches and individual Christians consider how to respond to the opportunities for ministry presented by AIDS, care should be taken not to underestimate the complexity of the challenge, the difficulty of the task, and the level of commitment necessary to initiate an adequate response. AIDS is a complicated medical disorder that manifests itself in a variety of illnesses having varying effects on the person diagnosed and on his or her loved ones. This means that in developing ministries, flexibility and responsiveness to individual differences are important. AIDS ministries may be more difficult to design and implement because the variations between situations require personalized attention. Finally, a high level of commitment is required to begin and sustain AIDS ministries because of the impediments and frustrations that attend them. In short, AIDS ministries should be undertaken by congregations and individuals who have their eyes open to the probable burdens and blessings associated with these activities.

Similarly, as AIDS ministries are being considered, the boundaries of concern should be generously drawn. People with AIDS-related diagnoses and their loved ones are obvious and compelling subjects of concern. But AIDS has a ripple effect, touching ever more lives. The popular

media, governmental, and scientific attention given to the
prevention and treatment of AIDS has made it a matter
of concern to almost everyone. As such, few people have
escaped the touch of AIDS. Unfortunately, some people
have been or are presently caught in its destructive grasp,
and ultimately few people will escape its touch entirely.
Thus, AIDS ministries should be open-ended as well as
open-eyed.

All ministries are related to faith commitments in two
ways.[1] First, what is believed about God, the mission of
the church, and discipleship influences the selection of
ministries, their interpretation, and their manner of implementation. It is also true that events and experiences
affect our beliefs about God, ecclesiology, and discipleship. For example, the appearance of AIDS prompted a
new examination of Christian teachings about illness and
outcast populations. This examination had two objectives:
(1) to determine how the resources of faith can incorpo-
rate AIDS into its worldview and (2) to determine how the
authorities of the faith inform and fashion the response of
the faithful to AIDS. Our study has led us to conclude that
the faithful are obligated to act compassionately toward
all people who are ill, without regard for their identity or
the way they contracted the disease, and that the faithful
have special obligations under God to befriend and defend
those who have few others to address their needs or advocate their cause. In sum, the church's response to AIDS
will reflect the extent to which it identifies itself with its
Lord, follows Jesus' teaching, and imitates his conduct.

The ministries proposed in this chapter reflect the authors' experience with people touched by AIDS directly
and indirectly, on the one hand, and their experience in
organizing and conducting ministries to these groups on
the other hand. The discussion ought not be understood
as a step-by-step recipe or a definitive guide to AIDS
ministries. Rather, it is intended to be programmatic, suggestive, and descriptive. This approach is required because
of the differences in needs and resources that exist between
congregations and the specific opportunities for ministry

in any given community. Thus, the applicability of any or all of the following proposals ultimately will have to be determined by individuals and congregations who feel called to be a compassionate and redeeming presence in the midst of the AIDS crisis.

General Prerequisites for Ministry

Ministering to people touched by AIDS differs in several ways from ministering to people with other illnesses. The objectives in both instances may be similar, but the negative moral attitudes, poor medical prognoses, and harsh social judgments associated with AIDS set it apart from other situations of ministry. As a result, before embarking on an AIDS ministry, three general prerequisites for ministry and three organizational recommendations warrant consideration.

Individual and Corporate Self-Examination

Being involved with people touched by AIDS can be a controversial activity. The fears evoked by the disease and the negative attitudes toward people who are at high risk (gay and bisexual men and IV drug users) can combine to become a significant barrier to ministry. This may be the case even though individuals and congregations may feel compassion for those who are suffering in this crisis. Some will hesitate to become involved, and some may refuse because of a concern not to offend people who oppose this ministry and to protect important relationships that might be jeopardized by unsympathetic friends. The risk to fellowship that an AIDS ministry may pose ought not be underestimated. The respective risks and benefits deserve consideration, but the final decision to embark upon an AIDS ministry should be guided by the imperatives of Christian discipleship. Clearly the perspective offered here is that the Christian mission authorizes and embraces ministry to people with AIDS. Yet such an undertaking may affect the fellowship of believers, and that fellowship deserves to be protected and preserved as much as possible, while being faithful to the Christian mission.

Initiating an AIDS ministry may first of all require courage. [2] The threat does not come from people with AIDS or related diagnoses. They do not represent a threat of infection as a result of casual contact—or even more intimate contact, provided that proper precautions are taken. Rather, people involved in AIDS ministries may require courage to deal with those who oppose that ministry. Criticism and withdrawal may result. Subtle and overt messages of disapproval may be encountered. The isolation and ostracism common to AIDS patients may be experienced by those who participate in hands-on ministries to these men, women, and children. Debates may develop about the type and means of ministry that are indicated by the AIDS crisis—should it be supportive or evangelistic? In short, the commitment to AIDS ministries may be tested severely during the planning and implementation phases.

The possible strain on fellowship may intensify as people with AIDS remain or become part of the corporate life of the congregation. Embracing people who are generally feared and disliked may be less threatening to fellowship as long as it is an activity outside the physical structure of the church. But if an AIDS ministry is to have maximum integrity it would seem to require a willingness to include in the multifaceted life of the congregation the people to whom ministry is offered. Restricting ministry to a home, hospital, or hospice setting is a signal that people suffering from AIDS are less valued and acceptable than people suffering from other illnesses. This sort of discrimination undercuts the proclamation of divine and human love implicit in an AIDS ministry. Redeeming love unites; it does not exclude or segregate. The discomfort or risk to fellowship that may accompany any innovative, pioneering, or controversial ministry may be intensified in the case of AIDS ministries.

The sentiments that arouse opposition to an AIDS ministry may be deeply ingrained and are not likely to be easily surmounted. Confronting reservations in a medically educated, socially unprejudiced, and theologically informed manner will require an openness of mind and heart. Agreeing to affirm mutual respect for the differing understandings and commitments of individuals and congregations may be a means by which diverse ministries may be undertaken and a harmonious fellowship maintained.

The second consideration is an assessment of how comfortable one is with illness, wasted bodies, anguish, death, and grief. People with AIDS tend to have repeated acute illnesses that result in an ever-increasing level of dependency. Their care can be very demanding. Care providers grow weary and frustrated as one acute illness ends and another soon appears. The physical and emotional toll is even greater for the ill person. The patient's loss of control over daily activity, environment, and body may be sudden or gradual. Whatever the speed, patients generally feel trapped in a process of irreversible debilitation and degeneration. Their bodies tend to waste away. Their anguish, anger, and grief tend to modulate as they adjust to the fact that neither they nor their physicians can control events.

People who enter this world to minister would be wise to anticipate this process. Not only should they imagine sojourning with one person and his or her loved ones through this course, they should anticipate repeating the cycle again and again at short intervals. A bond frequently develops between people, ill and well, who unite to combat AIDS and its devastating effects. Investments are made in one another. Commitments of care and personal presence are made and kept. Young men and women in their prime are pulled toward debilitation, dependency, indignity, and death. Being a part of this tragedy can be as exhausting as it can be rewarding.

Once acquainted with AIDS, one rarely fails to be moved by the suffering that surrounds it. Even people who are hostile toward high-risk populations or fearful of the disease often will respond compassionately in the face of such severe human pain and suffering. Moral condemnation and fear may remain intact, but empathy and sympathy usually move people to compassion and involvement. Suffering humanity, regardless of accompanying judgments of desert, can be a compelling force that draws even reluctant people into action. While a compassionate response, regardless of its source, is to be celebrated, it needs to be equal to the task. In practical terms, the extent and severity of disease and bodily destruction can be such that persons who wish to help can become immobilized. An inability to fulfill intentions may come from unavoidable unpleasant sights or a too intimate identification with the person. The would-be helper may turn away in horror or in fear of inflicting additional pain on a person who has suffered too much already. As AIDS ministries are contemplated, people intending a hands-on ministry ought to anticipate what surely lies ahead as a means to determine if they can bear the pain and still provide an effective ministry. An initial affirmative response ought not to be considered irrevocable. Though a person's fantasy about AIDS and its effects may be worse than the reality in some cases, in other cases the reality is far worse. Withdrawing is no disgrace, especially if persevering would be counterproductive for all concerned.

A third area of self-examination is one's willingness to be exposed to settings and lifestyles that are unfamiliar or even offensive. Some features of male homosexual culture, for example, may be interesting or they may be a significant barrier to ministry for people previously unaware of them.[3] The culture of IV drug users may engender a similar range of reactions.[4] It is important to remember, however, that meeting people in their own environment certifies declarations of concern and affirms their value under God. Ministry to people with AIDS entails entering into their experience, learning about them, loving them, and sharing their grief. In the process, friendships are forged, commitments are made, life is shared, and horizons are expanded. What was previously foreign may become familiar as a consequence of an AIDS ministry. Whether prior stereotypes or prejudices on either side are altered in the process appears less important on balance than the willingness to seek and sustain contact.

All people involved with AIDS should meet on the same level: one person loved by God meeting another person loved by God; one person of inestimable value to God meeting another person of inestimable value to God; one vulnerable and mortal person meeting another vulnerable and mortal person. This encounter of persons, not stereotypes, is essential to a valid and successful AIDS ministry. Condescension or self-righteousness on the part of God's people is contrary to the example of Jesus, and it is usually repulsive to the very people to whom ministry is offered. The object of God's people in ministries of compassion is to be a manifestation of God's love, implicitly inviting people to faith and obedience. There is no biblical warrant for abusing the weakness and vulnerability of persons. Jesus did not browbeat weakened people into declarations of faith. Even the "deathbed conversion" of the thief on the cross was a voluntary response to the love of God revealed in Jesus (Luke 23:39–43). Entering into the experience of others, as Jesus learned, may place one in uncomfortable or threatening surroundings. Nevertheless, the command to love one's neighbor contains no exceptions. And for the people of God, there are few more powerful expressions of love for God and neighbor than that of entering unconditionally into a neighbor's experience of pain and suffering.

A fourth area is one's capacity to separate compassion from condoning the conduct by which a person was infected with the AIDS virus. Some people may resist participating in supportive ministries because they do not wish their compassion to be interpreted as approving homosexual conduct, heterosexual marital infidelity, or IV drug use. These activities are widely condemned in church declarations and by individual Christians. Giving support to people who engage in these activities but who are now ill ought not be seen as an endorsement of their conduct. Christians who sincerely oppose smoking tobacco or alcohol consumption tend not to withdraw their support from people who become ill as a consequence of these lifestyles. In addition, the incidence of disease related to eating patterns and sedentary lifestyles appears even greater than the amount of disease related to tobacco and alcohol. Yet it is rare for Christians to turn away from people suffering from illnesses related to these activities out of fear that their presence and comforting ministries will be seen as condoning tobacco, alcohol, and food addiction. It may be that these latter "evils" have become domesticated over time and are now more socially tolerable, if not fully accepted, socially and religiously. People with diseases related to diet and "soft drug" addiction are not considered beyond the scope of Christian compassion.

People with AIDS as a consequence of socially and religiously disapproved behavior ought not to be seen as a separate category of ill person, unworthy of ministry because the conduct that contributed to their illness is opposed by a significant segment of the religious community. To withhold or withdraw ministry for this reason is inconsistent with the obligations to be faithful to those who are either ill or outcast.[5] Ministries of compassion are not necessarily indicative of one's moral opinion of a person or lifestyle, but such ministries are moral statements about the value of each person to God and to the community of faith. In this sense, AIDS ministries represent moral and theological understandings of duty and the value of persons. They do not, in and of themselves, constitute acceptance, tolerance, or advocacy of homosexuality, marital infidelity, or IV drug use. The behavior associated with the transmission of AIDS warrants consideration apart from the task of defining and fulfilling one's duties to sick, dying, and grieving persons. Unfortunately, it appears in the case of AIDS that negative moral judgments may distort our understandings of ministry, effectively blocking ministry to persons touched by AIDS. People disposed to participate in compassionate AIDS ministries should be able to separate in their own minds compassion from moral judgment. Similarly, they ought to recognize and be prepared to respond to the confusion of the two by other people.

A fifth area of self-examination before being involved in an AIDS ministry *is an assessment of the degree of commitment to the task.* The needs of each case may fluctuate greatly over short intervals of time. Ministering successfully in this situation requires individual and organizational flexibility, capacity to tolerate rapid changes, and an ability to persevere for a relatively long time. People who commit themselves to an AIDS ministry should be willing to be inconvenienced and to sacrifice personal interests for the needs of those served. The course of the disease and the level of dependency are not always predictable. Anticipating or expecting unforeseen requests for assistance may lessen the anger or frustration when they occur. Failing to respond to legitimate calls for help may intensify a patient's sense of being out of control, isolated, and abandoned. Loyalty to persons and keeping promises are important components for building secure relationships with people touched by AIDS. Alternately, the trust and confidence that persons with AIDS and their loved ones have in those who minister to them provide important bases for deepened relationships and expanded opportunities for ministry. Being clear in advance about the general type and number of ministries that may be requested allows people to determine whether their commitment to AIDS ministries is equal to the task.

The sixth area of self-examination is the availability of time. People with AIDS may feel that the church and Christians generally are unconcerned about them as persons or about their welfare. They often feel rejected and despised because of their sexuality, lifestyle, or disease. They probably have not felt welcomed in the life of most Christian churches. As a result, they have come to distrust a church that condemns them and Christians who insist that they change their sexual nature. Overtures by congregations to people with AIDS may be greeted with a degree of skepticism. The motives and objectives both may be questioned. Many outcast people feel initially that it is hypocritical of Christians to declare their love and offer comfort in situations of illness while being hostile or indifferent, at best, before the onset of a medical crisis. Overcoming this suspicion and accompanying reluctance to believe the honorable intentions of people committed to AIDS ministries requires patience, loyalty, and perseverance. An inordinate amount of time may be required both to initiate and sustain AIDS ministries. Working with the AIDS population is often an activity that cannot be predicted or scheduled. Ministries may occur at prearranged times and locations. They are equally likely to occur on request at inconvenient times and locations. People considering AIDS ministries should realize in advance that establishing quality relationships and providing quality ministries often requires many hours of preparation and activity.

The seventh area of self-examination requires an ability to maintain self-control, as is generally important for ministry to persons in crisis situations. People should anticipate that the activities undertaken will involve them in intimate, highly personal, and private situations. There must be a sufficient commitment to enable volunteers not to flee, and there must be a balancing objectivity that enables them to be effective. When this balance of commitment and objectivity is maintained, people are freed to minister, to be involved but not be immobilized, to feel but not decompensate.[6] Determining whether candidates for AIDS ministries have the necessary character and personality traits to attain this balance is largely a matter of self-examination and experience. An objective personal appraisal may be sufficient to identify people with the appropriate disposition and willingness. Actual ministry to people touched by AIDS either will confirm or invalidate this initial assessment. Undiscovered resources may emerge in the process of ministry. Similarly, the initial assessment of personal traits and skills may be found wanting when tested in actual ministry. Should this be the case, withdrawing from AIDS ministries, either from direct to indirect ministries or to total withdrawal, ought not to be seen as a defeat or embarrassment. More appropriately, this finding should be interpreted to indicate that one's gifts are better suited for alternate ministries. *The final area of self-examination builds upon positive responses to the preceding seven areas.* People who have the appropriate dispositions, traits, and opportunities to participate in AIDS ministries also need to be willing to be educated and trained for this specialized ministry. AIDS and its effects on people, both as a consequence of the disease itself and society's reaction to it, have created an unprecedented situation. Much is known and more is being learned.[7] Becoming informed about the destructive forces set in motion by HIV and how to respond in a healing, consoling, constructive manner are necessary conditions for embarking upon ministries to people touched by AIDS.

Education and Training

Being properly prepared can facilitate a competent and effective AIDS ministry. Education and training can take various forms, but they are indispensable. People who participate in AIDS ministries should be *learning as much as possible about the disease.* Learning about the AIDS virus and the means of its transmission should help to allay common fears and anxieties that surface as AIDS ministries are being planned. Distinguishing between the facts and myths about the routes of infection followed by the AIDS virus should help people feel comfortable about contact with people with AIDS and free them to minister confidently. In addition, knowledge of the common acute illnesses, treatments, and the general course of the syndrome can help people know what may happen and so formulate responses and ministries in advance of the need for them.

Learning about AIDS requires more than learning about the medical and physical facts. It means learning about the psychosocial aspects of the disease itself and the epidemic. The emotional, social, economic, and relational losses associated with AIDS can be as severe and destructive to the patient and to loved ones as the physical losses. People ministering to persons with AIDS should learn of thè emotional assaults, social reactions, economic costs, and individual rejections that may follow a diagnosis of AIDS. Being aware of these possibilities and their impact on the affected individuals should enhance a person's ability to understand the feelings of people bearing the stigma of AIDS. A better understanding, however, is not the only gain from becoming knowledgeable about the nonmedical aspects of AIDS. While cognitive awareness may inform and equip people involved in AIDS ministries, subjective or empathic knowledge contributes to a person's capacity to *feel and understand* what and how people touched by AIDS feel. Communicating, relating, experiencing, and ministering at this level may enrich the quality of the activity and contribute to its success. This is the level of mutual personal investment that, when achieved, creates interpersonal bonds sufficient to withstand the stresses and strains that inevitably develop.

Learning about the physical and psychosocial manifestations of AIDS involves *learning about people who are at high risk* for contracting the disease. It is well known that gay men and IV drug users are most likely to be infected by the AIDS virus and to become clinically ill as a result. The prospects for effective ministries are enhanced if the people seeking to minister become knowledgeable about male homosexuality, gay lifestyles, and the struggle of homosexual people for ecclesiastical, social, and legal equality.[8] Similarly, the phenomenon of drug abuse is complex, not easily explained or morally judged when considered comprehensively as both an individual activity and one that is culturally induced. Becoming familiar with relevant factual literature in both these areas should facilitate constructive interaction with these groups.[9] Learning about high-risk populations can be a means by which volunteers can assess their comfort level with either group before contact with them. Also, greater knowledge and understanding lessens the likelihood that people engaged in AIDS ministries will be surprised, shocked, or turned away by certain features or characteristics of either population.

A third component of the preparatory phase for AIDS ministries is *securing education and training in methods of pastoral care and ministry.* These activities are pastoral in the sense that they are supportive and nurturing, not that they are performed by ordained people. They are ministries of and by congregations. The duties of support and nurture belong to the laity as well as to those who are ordained. Just as ordained clergy typically are expected to be educated and trained in their profession before embarking upon it, people willing to provide AIDS ministries should be expected to have their gifts for ministry refined by special education and training that equip them for the task.[10] Among the skills that should be mastered at this point are the ability to listen, the ability to be nonjudgmental, the capacity to keep confidences, and the ability to persevere in the midst of hurt and grief. Finally, given the probable intensity of ministries to people with AIDS and their loved ones, appropriate oversight or supervision ought to be provided.[11] Learning to minister under supervision enables an observer to spot emerging problems and to provide counsel about how to avoid or minimize them. In addition, the supervisor can provide support, nurture, and consolation to the people engaged in hands-on ministries. The stress, hurt, and grief that are typical features of AIDS ministries can be addressed by the supervisor in order to meet the needs of the people ministering and to guard against burnout.

In addition to learning how to provide emotional and spiritual care to the sick and their loved ones, people participating in hands-on AIDS ministries may need help in *learning how to perform unskilled or semiskilled nursing tasks.* These procedures may include moving a bed-bound patient, positioning a patient in bed for comfort, changing diapers on adults, oral care, and feeding, watering, cleaning, and medicating patients (orally and via IV lines).

Providing these types of care may give relief to the primary caregivers. They are tangible expressions of concern. They are evidence that inhibiting fears have been overcome.

Continuing one's education is the fifth component. Knowledge about the disease and its impact is constantly growing. Participants in AIDS ministries cannot be expected to become or remain experts on the AIDS crisis or any single aspect of it. Nevertheless, they should be alert to news reports about the disease, its treatment, and societal responses to it. These subjects often are topics of discussion during visits. Staying aware of these developments indicates a high level of interest and facilitates interaction. In addition, this knowledge can be called upon to teach people the facts about AIDS, especially the means and risks of transmission of the virus. Workshops and seminars with appropriate leadership can help achieve this objective. Similar sessions focusing on increasing knowledge about ministry and gaining or improving ministering skills also would be appropriate.

These five aspects of preparatory education and training are separately and jointly intended to enhance the competence and self-confidence of participants in AIDS ministries. By establishing an effective training program, a means is provided by which new participants can be incorporated into ongoing activities. Veteran members can keep their knowledge current and their ministering skills sharply honed. With adequate preparation and opportunities for continued education, people involved in AIDS ministries should be better able to respond creatively and confidently to unexpected challenges.

Clarity of Purpose

AIDS ministries are primarily ministries of support, nurture, and consolation. They are not primarily evangelistic ministries in the sense of pressure to convert to a particular faith or morality. To view evangelism as the primary or sole objective of ministry to people with AIDS is to misunderstand ministry and probably will be counterproductive with the targeted audience. Authentic ministry involves the free gift of self to others, echoing God's free gift of the divine self to humanity. It involves establishing knowing and sharing relationships characterized biblically as loving one's neighbor. This and only this is the formal end of ministry. People, especially in evangelical churches, often are inclined to understand all ministries to be aimed ultimately at "saving the lost." But "saving" people is not the business of human beings. It is a task beyond their power. "Saving" people, it should be remembered, is God's business.[12] Thus, the purpose for all ministry, including AIDS ministry, is to represent God's love for all humanity, without condition, and to embody and express that love in all human relationships.

Doors are likely to be closed quickly to well-meaning people who approach men and women caught in the crisis of AIDS with declarations of their sin and need for repentance. This approach seems to some people as most properly directed toward gay or bisexual men caught in the AIDS crisis. Their "sin" is said to be what they do sexually and who they discover themselves to be: homosexual. Intravenous drug users are said to be morally culpable for their actions only, not for who they are as sexual beings, provided that they are heterosexual. In both groups, however, approaches by Christians that are in reality reproaches tend to be rejected. The prospect for relationship is significantly lessened when the first priority is seen to be that of convincing people that they are evil, in the case of nonheterosexual men with AIDS. Further, ministries to drug users conditioned on changed behavior are likely to be exercises in frustration, since drug addictions tend not to be remedied by acts of will alone.

In order for AIDS ministries to be initiated and to mature, contact with affected individuals needs to be maintained. People with AIDS are more likely to allow others to sojourn with them when they feel accepted by and acceptable to people who want to help. As everyone becomes more confident that the expressed concern is genuine and masks no coercive agenda, trust develops. Patients and their loved ones may begin to feel comfortable enough to initiate discussions about their spiritual concerns, to which people involved in AIDS ministries legitimately may respond. Setting the spiritual agenda in AIDS ministries is a task to be performed by the recipients of these ministries, not the people providing them. Once raised, these subjects can be addressed in a constructive, redemptive, gentle manner, affirming to all that God's invitation to fellowship is constant and that God's love excludes no one. It seems more important, in these situations, to manifest divine and human love that encourages a turning to God than to attempt to require that a person's relationship with God conform to any particular confession or morality.

The distinctive aspect of the AIDS ministries envisaged here is the loving care offered by God's people, not the tasks that are performed. Almost all services proposed in this chapter, except for sacraments and other religious rites, can be performed competently by non-Christians. It is this feature of the church's ministry in the AIDS crisis that distinguishes it from the services provided by governments and secular agencies. The church's ministry, without fanfare and without coercion, ought to be a humble act of service following the example of its servant Lord. The church's healing presence demonstrates God's compassion and concern for all people burdened as a consequence of AIDS. Thus, AIDS ministries are to be supportive, compassionate, consoling, and reconciling. They manifest God's involvement and call all segments of society to a godly response.

Organizational Recommendations

Parish-Based Care

The care of sick and suffering people is a duty of God's people. Although the institution of the church may sponsor or operate facilities and conduct programs through which care is provided, the actual ministry, in whatever form it takes, is performed by individuals. Church-related hospitals, nursing homes, hospices, and residences are laudable activities. However, these operations do not satisfy the obligation of individual Christians to address the needs of people coping with illness and the impact of death. Congregants routinely express concern and provide care for fellow congregants in crisis. The provision of similar ministries to persons outside congregational membership is less common, except through the caring institutions founded and operated by parishes and denominations. Yet in the case of AIDS, the opportunities for ministry are greater outside the confines of these church-sponsored institutions because efforts are made to maintain AIDS patients in their homes as much as possible. Hospitalization, though frequent in some cases, tends to be short-term. It is difficult to create and sustain relationships when contact is restricted to periods of institutional care. These opportunities for ministry ought not to be overlooked. But with a chronic degenerative disease like AIDS, the needs of the people afflicted persist and tend to increase between times in the hospital. Therefore, the prospect for enduring and effective ministries increases if these ministries are parish-based rather than hospital-based.

As noted, ministering in a comprehensive manner to people with AIDS may require a large investment of time and energy. In addition, the needs of affected individuals can be so numerous and demanding that a single patient and his or her loved ones may require the ministries of many people. This situation seems to be best addressed by ministry teams formed within single parishes.[13] A team approach can draw upon the diverse expertise within a parish, provide for efficient coordination of activities, enhance communication within the team and with the patient, make possible a division of labor, and facilitate mutual care for the team members. Matching a parish-based team with a patient also encourages enduring contact and

bonding between team members and the patient and between the parish and the patient. The results this approach
wants to achieve are relationships of deeper quality, mutual commitments of greater intensity, and deeper trust
and concern. This sort of team ministry may make it possible for a
patient and loved ones to establish rapport with one or
more team members. Further, the affected individuals
may develop a sense of belonging to a particular family
of faith, frequently resulting in a congregation's becoming a surrogate "home church" for loved ones who have
come a long distance to remain with a patient during his
or her illness. This seems most likely when the ministry
team and affected people are of the same denomination.
Lastly, a team ministry is advisable, because realistically
only a limited number of people in a parish will feel led
to participate in AIDS ministries. Each will possess certain gifts that deserve to be used efficiently and effectively. A team approach should allow for a continuing
and coordinated ministry. Thus, a self-contained unit
consisting of people with a common identity, mission,
and parish base offers the best likelihood for a successful
ministry.

Interfaith Ministries

The opportunities for ministry occasioned by AIDS in
locations where there are many cases tend to be greater
than any single parish or denomination can effectively
provide. AIDS affects people in all religious traditions,
and therefore all religious traditions have a responsibility
to conduct AIDS ministries. An interfaith AIDS ministry
can provide a coordinated program through which faith
groups support and complement each other. Such a structure also enables a coordinating staff to match patients and
families with a parish team of their own faith.

However, such matching is not always required. Some
people needing help prefer that it come from a denomina-

tion other than their own, particularly if their denomination is known to be unsympathetic to homosexual people or to the plight of people with AIDS. In our experience it has proved difficult to organize an AIDS ministry that is truly ecumenical, involving individuals from several denominations in a patient-directed team. Nevertheless, the appearance and spread of AIDS is creating a growing need and opportunity for ministry that transcends traditional denominational boundaries, ideally stimulating on some levels a joint response by religious bodies. Judaism and Christianity have a common concern for ill, suffering, and bereaved persons. AIDS is an area where this concern can lead to cooperation without compromising theological distinctives or violating polity. Joint educational and service projects may be possible with AIDS but perhaps not with many other issues. In addition, if parishes and church bodies sponsor some joint activities in response to AIDS, there is an opportunity for each to learn about the other: more particularly, what they share that brought them together on this issue and the differences that inhibit cooperation in other areas.

The final reason why parish-based AIDS ministries ought to be interfaith is geographic. People touched by AIDS can be found nearly everywhere. Although people with confirmed diagnoses are concentrated in metropolitan areas, they and their loved ones live in all neighborhoods. It is unrealistic to conclude that parishes in neighborhoods with a large number of high-risk people are the only ones facing the problem, or that they are able to address all the needs. The people who need AIDS-related ministries are dispersed throughout the city limits and across the countryside. Parishes next to treatment institutions or in high-risk population areas cannot effectively minister to loved ones in other areas of the city or country. Moreover, it is important that parishes conducting AIDS ministries let their work be widely known. It does little good to have a ministry that is not known to people who would benefit from it. Publicizing the parish's stand on this issue and the ministries offered is essential. Further, referral is facilitated when parishes are aware of resources available in other parishes.

Networks

Publicizing a parish's AIDS ministries is important for reasons other than interparish referral. People desiring AIDS ministries need to know where they can turn for support, nurture, and consolation. Self-referral to a parish is one means to initiate a relationship with people coping with AIDS. An equally important means is by referral relationships with health care personnel, relevant agencies, and AIDS support organizations. There ought to be a spirit of cooperation among resource agencies grounded in a common concern for how best to serve the needs of people touched by AIDS. The limited governmental response to AIDS means that much of the psychosocial and physical and nearly all the spiritual care of this population falls to volunteer organizations, including the church. Competition and unnecessary duplication of scarce resources ought to be avoided. If interested persons and agencies cooperate in every way possible, supplementing the resources that each provides, this network will make it more possible to provide appropriate care in an efficient and effective manner.

In our experience, patients and loved ones are hesitant to ask churches and church people for help. They anticipate a hostile, condemning, or indifferent response. Secular and governmental agencies are seen as their primary hope for assistance and as forums where they will be received with some degree of respect. Whether this perception is valid depends on the agency and personnel involved. Nevertheless, because religious communities, intentionally or unintentionally, have caused people at high risk to feel unwelcome when diagnosed as having AIDS or a related disorder, they do not see the church as a resource, feeling it does not care about them or their struggle to survive. If contact is to be made with these distrustful individuals, it may need to be facilitated by secular agencies. When a parish AIDS ministry team and a patient are matched, the process of creating trust, of discrediting false perceptions with regard to that particular parish, and of providing supportive ministries may begin. Networking with secular and religious agencies, therefore, tends to be crucial in many instances. Without a reliable network, available ministries may not be performed and all concerned will be worse off.

A final possible good to be realized from networking relates to public attitudes. When ecclesiastical and secular institutions can embrace a single position and coordinate resources to address a family of needs, they can make a powerful prophetic statement. In the case of AIDS, a cooperative response signals that AIDS is a public health crisis rather than a moral issue. It is an occasion for mobilizing a coordinated, comprehensive response, not an occasion to point fingers of blame and abdicate responsibility. It is a crisis that calls for a benevolent and compassionate attitude toward suffering people from all sectors of the community. By responding in a praiseworthy manner, secular and religious institutions can model the attitude and behavior most appropriate to the needs of all concerned. By acting compassionately and responsibly, religious and secular agencies and officials can help all of society to make a reasoned, redemptive, humane response.

Sustaining Ministries

AIDS ministries are termed sustaining ministries because they inform, affirm, and support persons. They promote certain goods and values in the midst of a situation of significant loss. These ministries are multidirectional and serve a variety of ends. They are realistic, responsive to the needs arising from the crisis of AIDS, appropriate to the mission of God's people, and representative of a contemporary interpretation of the command to love one's neighbor. The types of ministries that follow have as their focus people presently touched directly by AIDS, the church's integrity, and the character of the society within which the church exists. In short, when seen as a whole and understood theologically, AIDS ministries have a prophetic, priestly, and servant character reflecting a concern for the well-being of individual persons, the church itself, and the social order.[14]

Education

Providing factual information about the extent of suffering engendered by AIDS is one way to combat fear, indifference, and hostility. There is resistance to learning about AIDS, both in society at large and within congregations. This may be related to the convergence of two taboos in the present public health crisis—sex and death.[15] Neither topic is usually discussed in polite circles. Sex and death denote powerful, awe-inspiring forces of generation and destruction. They attract and repel. They are clothed in mystery. Everyone is aware of them, but no one seems fully to understand them. They are linked in biblical myth to explain theologically the nature of the human condition. And both are associated with God's displeasure with humanity's exercise of freedom.[16]

Although sex and death are seen in scientific communities as legitimate subjects for analysis, in religious and nonscientific circles there is a tendency to regard both subjects and the phenomena related to them as off limits. Their mysterious nature is to remain intact. Since they are related to God's judgment, discussion of either except in approved ways is to be avoided. Thus, AIDS incorporates two taboos by being sexually transmitted and by being fatal. The situation currently is compounded further by its association in developed Western countries with another taboo—male homosexual conduct. The taboos associated with AIDS combine to form an effective barrier to educating church people and the public about the disease and the suffering it causes. The disease has been portrayed as additional evidence of God's anger over the violation of taboos and rules of conduct. Rather than being a party to these violations and risking a further outpouring of God's wrath, people tend to avoid education about AIDS. Yet education about how to prevent the spread of the AIDS virus is presently the best hope of limiting its destructive effect. And finally, putting a personal face on the pain and suffering caused by AIDS may be the most effective way to generate an informed, compassionate response.

The losses AIDS causes and the opportunities for ministry it creates cannot be ignored. It seems advisable to face them now while the human toll is comparatively limited, rather than later when the intensity of human suffering will have increased manyfold. In fact, becoming aware of the probable magnitude of the crisis may motivate people to prepare now to meet current and projected needs. The church classroom and the pulpit are appropriate forums in which to provide facts about AIDS and summon a compassionate response. The church classroom seems better suited, however, for examining several topics in detail and developing a comprehensive understanding of AIDS and the church's role in the epidemic.

The Church Classroom. The first obvious area of education is the disease itself. Print, videotape, and personal resources increasingly are available to provide people with a factual, understandable orientation to AIDS.[17] Sessions directed toward this end should include information on the AIDS virus, means of transmission, preventive measures, physiological tests for infection, symptoms of infection, effect of the virus on the body's immune system, secondary complications, and precautions to take when ministering to infected persons.

A second general subject of study is high-risk behavior patterns. Learning about AIDS presents an opportunity to provide accurate information about human sexuality and drug addiction in a nonprejudicial manner. The facts regarding the risks for infection during heterosexual and homosexual activity may be presented in a candid, unemotional, nonsensational manner. What is known about the etiology of sexual identity, sex roles, and sexual prefer-

ences could be communicated apart from moral judgments about any specific form of sexual activity. An important by-product of such a candid, factual presentation
regarding the sexual transmission of the AIDS virus
would be correcting the mistaken perception that AIDS is
a gay disease. Similarly, the psychological and social factors that contribute to drug abuse, promiscuity, and infidelity could be examined.

This two-pronged study of high-risk behavior could result in a better understanding of these issues and a decreased tendency to "blame the victim" of AIDS for his
or her distress. In short, all the factors that have had a role
in the rapid spread of the AIDS virus might be perceived.
So understood, partial responsibility for the AIDS crisis
rests upon society and its component institutions, as well
as upon individuals who knowingly and needlessly have
exposed themselves or others to infection.[18] By seeing that
AIDS is not the fault of any particular group of persons,
perhaps people will hesitate to scapegoat a particular
group for this evil. And finally, perhaps we can resist the
urge to use AIDS to frighten or coerce people to deny their
sexual identity or to adopt a particular lifestyle or morality. Decisions about these matters ought to be made on the
merits of the relevant arguments, not because of the association of a disease with a particular sexual practice or
behavior. Thus, if moral judgments are to be part of educational programs on AIDS, these judgments should be
properly based and directed fairly toward relevant persons, groups, institutions, and society, as well as the original high-risk populations.

A third subject for inquiry and reflection is the nature
of the human condition as vulnerable, finite, and mortal.
The world is filled with risks. Each day people die as a
result of disease, accident, war, social injustice, and homi-
cide. Other threats may not be lethal but nonetheless are
disruptive and painful. Illness, trauma, injury, hunger,
and assault impair and inconvenience people every day.
Although the possibility of injury or death is known, most
people go about their daily affairs in a prudent manner.

They are not paralyzed by the prospect of harm that might befall them. Apparently people consciously or subconsciously calculate the relative risks and goods associated with different activities and decide to act or not to act. Most people obviously conclude that the risk of falling in the shower is outweighed by the good of having a clean body. The good of visiting with a friend outweighs the risks of the drive to the friend's residence. The good of not developing mumps is greater than the risk associated with vaccination. People live as if the risks of daily living will never touch them. The absence of guarantees that nothing will happen does not stop most people from functioning in a productive and healthy manner.

Some people have attempted to justify their abandonment of people with AIDS by citing the absence of a guarantee that casual contact with infected persons is totally risk-free. Reputable physicians and scientists cannot say this with absolute certainty. They can, however, assure people that, on the basis of the extensive evidence gathered to date, casual contact does not constitute a risk of infection. The question to be asked in classes on the human condition is whether the good associated with a believer's duty toward sick and suffering people is not greater than the risk to one's welfare that may be attached to fulfilling that duty. In other words, Christians should consider the costs of discipleship and their willingness to incur those costs. People ought to understand that being a Christian may subject them to human opposition or place them in situations of possible danger. Accepting vulnerability, finitude, and mortality as inescapable features of human existence is a first step toward living freely and fully. When people are unwilling or unable to cope with these facts they tend to be enslaved by fear, incapable of entering relationships or participating in normal human activities. Yet Christian faith affirms that love casts out fear and propels people into relationships. Living lovingly does not mean ignoring risks. Rather, it means placing them in perspective, and acting prudently. The needs of others must not be ignored.

Making sense of vulnerability and mortality involves a consideration of God's loving will for humanity and the manner of God's involvement in history.[19] These are important subjects that warrant careful study. They are relevant to the AIDS epidemic because of the claim that AIDS is God's punishment on homosexual men and the nation that tolerates them. This claim asserts that there is a connection between the circumstances or fate of a person or society and God's evaluation of that person or society. This is a disputable claim that implicitly sanctions abandoning sick and suffering people or engenders hostility toward them as an extension of God's displeasure, wrath, or judgment. Yet, as demonstrated in chapters 3 and 4, this reasoning and conclusion is contrary to the witness of scripture regarding a believer's duty toward the sick and the value of the poor to God. If courses, lectures, or discussions about these matters are theologically instructive, they will help people understand and respond to AIDS.

A fourth topic of study is the healing ministry of Jesus and its continuation by the church. A review of the Gospels and of church history should help people to understand AIDS as simply another illness, albeit devastating, to which the people of God are obliged to respond creatively, in a compassionate and supportive manner. When seen in this perspective, AIDS ceases to be an occasion for condemnation and becomes an opportunity to represent and actualize God's love for suffering humanity. AIDS, therefore, challenges the church to claim its identity, to be faithful to its heritage, and to follow the example of its Lord. AIDS provides the people of God with an opportunity to formulate and implement ministries that are responsive to the specific needs of people touched by a new and destructive disease.

The Pulpit. Becoming educated about AIDS, placing it in theological perspective, and discerning the church's obligations to the men, women, and children who are touched by it are activities not limited to the church classroom. Education also is a function of the pulpit ministry.

Pastors and preachers can heighten a congregation's awareness of the suffering, needs, and opportunities for ministry that AIDS patients present by referring to them in intercessory prayers and sermons. Pastors can remind the congregation that they are called to be a servant people serving a servant Lord. Sermons can help people understand what servant ministry means and what obedience to the love command requires. In addition, sermons on the inclusive nature of God's love, God's presence in the midst of human suffering, corporate understanding of human well-being, and God as hope and refuge can influence attitudes and shape responses. Finally, pastors can proclaim that at the center of the gospel there is a divine call for reconciliation between God and humanity and between mutually estranged human beings. Such reconciliation could be exemplified in a congregation's response to AIDS. Parishioners could be reminded that in the life and death of Jesus a new way of reconciliation was established.

Spiritual and Sacramental Ministries

The second type of sustaining ministry is directed more toward people struggling with AIDS than toward the church itself, as in the educational ministries just proposed. Spiritual and sacramental ministries are meaningful ways to express God's and the church's concern for people in the present crisis. Intercessory prayers and healing rites communicate a human and divine concern for the physical and emotional well-being of the sick. Rites of baptism, communion, and participation in worship signify that the person with AIDS is a member of the family of faith. Supportive and compassionate ministries (pastoral care) validate and extend what these practices symbolize: that a person with AIDS and his or her loved ones are not abandoned by God's people in a time of crisis. Finally, funeral, burial, and memorial services provide hope to the bereaved and signify that the care and concern for the one who is dead extends beyond life. These spiritual and sacramental ministries can comfort people in distress and set an example for society to emulate.

Physical Assistance

The physical needs of people with AIDS or related diagnoses can vary between patients and fluctuate for an individual patient. The physical and monetary losses that characterize AIDS often create needs that congregations can meet. Numerous types of assistance can be organized and provided: preparation of meals, food pantry supplies, help in performing activities of daily living (e.g., dressing, bath, toilet), housecleaning, shopping, transportation, housing, financial subsidy, unskilled nursing care, relieving primary caregiver, home hospice care, inpatient hospice, and assistance to visiting family and friends. These ministries, when performed in a sensitive and effective manner, can significantly improve a patient's quality of life. They are means by which relationships with patients can be initiated and sustained. Thus these ministries benefit patients and enable the people of God to fulfill their calling.

Emotional Support

The physical losses that require supplementing are paralleled by emotional stresses. Feelings of abandonment, loneliness, and loss of self-esteem can be alleviated by expressions of concern and commitment through regular visits and phone calls. Separate support groups can be organized for patients, families (including lovers), clinicians, friends, and the worried well. These groups should be led by properly trained, adequately informed, and appropriately certified professionals. Groups that are heterogeneous, open to anyone with a concern or need, also can be a valuable source of emotional support. Finally, the experience of bereavement following an AIDS death tends to be different from common bereavement, because the cause of death may be kept secret or misrepresented. The process of catharsis and healing may be frustrated as a consequence. Bereavement groups restricted to these people may provide a safe haven where their specific and special feelings can be aired and their concerns addressed.

An area of emotional support that ought not be neglected is the care of the ministry team in a parish. As indicated above, AIDS ministries ought to be properly supervised. The intensity of these ministries can inflict a heavy toll on the people who provide them. An objective supervisor should be able to identify or foresee potential problems and act quickly to avoid them. Further, the emotional or spiritual needs of the team or its individual members may be addressed by a trained supervisor. It is important to remember that the caregivers probably will themselves require care because of the emotional assaults they sustain in the process of ministering in the AIDS crisis. The ability of team members properly to minister over the long term may depend on this type of resource's being available.

Social and Political Leadership

The church can provide moral leadership to society by formulating and implementing a compassionate response to AIDS.[20] This prophetic ministry can provide legal assistance to patients whose rights are being denied by employers, landlords, insurers, medical institutions, or governments. The church through its officials can articulate, advance, and defend the claims of people touched by AIDS for social services and for personal respect. Stigmatization and discrimination wherever found should be denounced. Government, at all levels, should not be allowed to be unchallenged in its failure to foster an attitude of compassion, conduct research, provide therapy, and protect the rights of patients. Political leaders should be subject to a similar scrutiny. Indifference, prejudice, discrimination, and hatred should be identified and condemned. Finally, claims that people with AIDS deserve their fate should be discredited, because they are mistaken and because they undermine simple decency and compassion. In order for the prophetic voice of the church to have credibility it must express justice and compassion in its response to AIDS. By so doing, the church is faithful to its identity and mission. And moreover, the church sets an example for other segments of society to follow.

These types of ministries and specific proposals are suggestive of what the church and God's people can do to fulfill their calling and to lessen the suffering caused by AIDS. Individually and collectively, AIDS ministries ought to be redemptive and prophetic, modeling an attitude that performs a teaching and healing function in society.

More specifically, AIDS ministries serve a variety of ends consistent with the gospel.

They embody the good news that all persons are valued by God and God's people. They are indications of care and concern for sick, suffering, and bereaved people. They are evidence of God's continued commitment to people abandoned or cast out in society. They represent God's will that the burden of oppression be lifted in whatever form it is found.

They are directed toward the relief of suffering and anguish. The church's healing presence in the midst of the AIDS crisis is a reminder that God is present to those who suffer. God's participation through the agency of the institutional church and of individual Christians ought to summon others to share in the work of countering the loneliness, isolation, stigma, and fear that too often are the only companions of people touched by AIDS. In short, the church's passive and active presence can sustain and heal, even in situations where physical cure is presently not available.

They are faithful to the church's identity and mission. The people of God are a servant people. By definition, they cannot neglect the needs of others. In this sense the church, in order to be true to itself and its Lord, needs people with AIDS more than people with AIDS need the church.

They are redemptive in form and function. AIDS ministries by their existence and performance weaken the barriers of prejudice, fear, suspicion, and hatred that separate people. They are testimony to God's inclusive love. They affirm the value of all persons to God.

They promote understanding and mutual respect between estranged groups. The church and people with AIDS are drawn into relationship because of their need for each other. Because of their respective need to give and receive help, the church and estranged populations (such as gay men, bisexual men, and IV drug users) have an opportunity to learn about, help, and develop respect for each other.

They enrich the lives of the people who serve and who are served. AIDS ministries seem to verify the claim that one gains life by spending it on others. The investment of life moves in two directions, each person investing in the life of the other. The tragic difference with AIDS is that one person will survive and the other will not. Yet each person is enriched as a result of the relationship.

Finally, they heal. Participants in AIDS ministries naturally hope that a cure soon will be found, but the absence of a cure ought not suggest that all healing is beyond reach. The healing that can occur is of indifference, mistrust, anger, hatred, prejudice, ignorance, callousness, and estrangement wherever and in whomever they are found. Such healing is likely when people, regardless of their differences, are willing to affirm each other's inherent value and dignity. This sort of healing is possible when each is willing to risk loving the other.

6

Concluding Reflections

The underlying theme of this book is simple. People with AIDS, their family members, and friends have a claim on church and synagogue simply by virtue of their plight. Perhaps there was a touch of irony in Jesus' voice as he challenged both his close friends and the Jewish religious leaders regarding their public behavior. To his friends and the curious crowd he presented the case for a quality of love that supersedes mere keeping of the technical rules. The forefathers were told to love their neighbors, but there is a higher order of relationship. We are to love our enemies and pray for our persecutors. *Only* by living in accordance with this "new" commandment can we be children of God. Jesus chided his listeners: If we love only those who love us, surely we would not look for any reward (for doing what is customary and expected). *Surely the tax gatherers do as much!* And if you greet only your brothers, what is extraordinary about that? Again Jesus observes, *even the heathen do as much!* The standard for relationship Jesus sets for his disciples is the example of God: "There must be no limit to your goodness, as your heavenly Father's goodness knows no bounds" (Matt. 5:48).

We may twist uncomfortably at such words. We may shrug them off as hyperbole, ideals surely not meant to be taken seriously. But Jesus does not leave us much room to wriggle. The message is hammered home at every opportunity, in stark language and with a piercing look. To the naive, he retorts that the Son of Man has nowhere to lay his head. The person who decides to follow him had better count the cost, because the going may get rough (Matt. 5:20; Luke 14:25–35). Indeed, Luke (14:26, 33) records Jesus' warning to his followers, "If anyone comes to me and does not hate his father and mother, wife and children, brothers and sisters, even his own life, he cannot be a disciple of mine. . . . None of you can be a disciple of mine without parting with all his possessions." Then comes the thundering warning: "Salt is a good thing; but if salt itself becomes tasteless . . . it is useless either on the land or on the dung-heap: it can only be thrown away. If you have ears to hear, then hear" (vs. 34–35). To the hesitant, he replied, "Follow me, and leave the dead to bury their dead" (Matt. 8:22), and "No one who sets his hand to the plough and then keeps looking back is fit for the kingdom of God" (Luke 9:62).

This unswerving commitment is required by the importance of the task to which Jesus' disciples are called: "You must go and announce the kingdom of God" (Luke 9:60). The apostles understood the intention of the call to announce the kingdom which would be manifested as they preached the good news and healed the sick and disabled. They knew the risk, for a follower must always be ready to take up his or her cross (e.g., Matt. 16:24) and walk in Christ's footsteps (Matt. 10:38; Luke 14:27).

The scriptures declare unambiguously that God looks with anger upon indifference to suffering, abuse of the weak, and abuse of privilege at the expense of the poor. God's feelings about these matters were expressed by the prophets. Isaiah, speaking to the nation, declared:

> Shame on you! you who make unjust laws
> and publish burdensome decrees,
> depriving the poor of justice,
> robbing the weakest of my people of their rights,

despoiling the widow and plundering the orphan.
What will you do when called to account,
when ruin from afar confronts you?
To whom will you flee for help
and where will you leave your children,
so that they do not cower before the gaoler
or fall by the executioner's hand?
For all this his anger has not turned back,
and his hand is stretched out still.

Isaiah 10:1–4

Jeremiah echoed Isaiah's words:

But your wrongdoing has upset nature's order,
and your sins have kept from you her kindly gifts.
For among my people there are wicked men,
who lay snares like a fowler's net
and set deadly traps to catch men.
Their houses are full of fraud,
as a cage is full of birds.
They grow rich and grand,
bloated and rancorous;
their thoughts are all of evil,
and they refuse to do justice,
the claims of the orphan they do not put right
nor do they grant justice to the poor.
Shall I not punish them for this?
says the LORD;
shall I not take vengeance
on such a people?

Jeremiah 5:25–29

The prophets' message (see also Hosea 4:2–3; Amos 2:6–7; 4:1–3; Micah 6:9–15) is echoed by Jesus. Since the care and nurture of the poor was mandated by Torah, Jesus' general warning clearly applies: If one sets aside "even the least of the Law's demands, and teaches others to do the same, he [or she] will have the lowest place in the kingdom of Heaven" (Matt. 5:19). But Jesus was even more specific, as seen in Matthew's record of Jesus cleansing the temple (21:12–13). It was not merely the commercial enterprise that was under judgment; the money-changers and the dealers in pigeons customarily used their privileges to enrich themselves at the expense of the poor who came to worship. In his confrontation with the doctors of the Law and the Pharisees (Matt. 23:1–36), he accuses the rulers of overlooking the "weightier" demands of the Law—justice, mercy, and good faith (v. 23). Especially in the parable of the last judgment (Matt. 25:31–46), he rebukes those who failed to exercise loving care toward the poor. The message, once again, is stark and unrelenting. We are expected to do for others what God has done for us. And, just as clearly, we will not be called into God's presence unless we show compassion to the excluded and welcome them into the community of God's people.

Jesus did not merely greet sinners. He included them with other social groups to whom the gospel applied equally, invited them into the kingdom, and encouraged his followers to do likewise. He engaged in intimate actions which dramatized his personal concern for them. He searched for them (Luke 14:23) and welcomed both table fellowship and physical touch. The scriptural image of hospitality played an important part in Jesus' teaching. Through accepting those who were "different," he declared clean what others regarded as defiled. Mere hospitality takes seriously the differences, the "otherness" that separates people from one another. But the metaphor invites us to supersede those differences in order to achieve a higher end: recognition and acceptance of our common humanity as children of God.

Jesus' inclusion of outcasts, those who are "different," is embedded in references to the poor generally. In the Beatitudes, Jesus used the words "the poor" and "those who mourn" in their original sense. They are those who expect nothing from society and thus expect everything from God. The poor do not fit into the structure of the world and therefore are rejected by it. The Beatitudes alert God's people that the weak and powerless are unable to obtain recognition from society; therefore, the people of God must act for them. The situation of people who are at the limits of human existence is not to be glorified in itself. Misery and poverty mean distress and torture, just as do blindness, lameness, leprosy—and the prospect of death from AIDS.

The message of the Jewish and Christian scriptures is that God comes near to give counsel and to reprove, but also to call people to a loving relationship. The Old Testament offers many images of God's initiative: to Abraham (Gen. 18:1–15); to Jacob (Gen. 28:13); to Moses (Ex. 3:2); to Samuel (1 Sam. 3:4–14); to Elijah (1 Kings 19:9–18); to Isaiah (Isa. 6:1–13); to Ezekiel (Ezek. 2:1–3:11). God not only reveals the divine presence to the commissioned representatives—kings and prophets—but, through them, continually both reassures and reprimands the entire nation. The New Testament images continue this emphasis, as the writer of the letter to the Hebrews testifies (1:1–3). God has taken the initiative to show the divine nature and purpose to humanity and to call humanity into fellowship with God, a theme reflected, for example, in the kingdom parables relating to invitations to the king's feast (e.g., Matt. 22:1–14). The implications are clear for God's people in the midst of the AIDS crisis: There is an urgency to the task of finding the outcasts and embodying God's invitation to them. But with that task comes a warning: The despised (to Jesus' hearers, "tax-gatherers and prostitutes") are entering the kingdom of God ahead of those who expected to occupy the places of honor (Matt. 21:31). God's people are sent as servants to summon and offer hospitality to people excluded by society, inviting them to participate in the joy of God's kingdom. For in this royal priesthood, this dedicated nation, all are welcome.

The people of God are called, therefore, to be a community which welcomes "the poor" and treats them as full members of the community. When love for God is manifested through love for people, as well as for the world which also is an object of God's love, the church becomes a sign to the world, signifying that community which is God's gift to all people. Each member of the community is to be a manifestation of that community into which other people may choose to enter. Members of God's community are called to express love to the neighbor, to welcome the stranger, to speak comfort to the poor, and all in the context of announcing the kingdom of God and manifesting its presence and activity.

Forming and sustaining God's community is an adventure that requires courage and hope. As a community of faith, the church is summoned to live by values other than those that predominate in the world. Society *beyond* the church may choose to be blind and deaf to the needs of people whom it either has, or wishes it could, cast aside—though there are many heartwarming instances of citizens who manifest concern and compassion for the outcast, including people with AIDS. But the church does not have an option to be uninvolved. It is a community that must be characterized by a compassion which seeks out the outcast as the objects of its love.

This Christian courage includes, but is not limited to, the readiness to take the next step, to become involved in ministry to people with AIDS. Health and physical risks are minimal. Courage is required to face with the patient or family the imminence of death, the wasting effects of infection, the questions about the meaning of life, and the meaning of this disease in particular. Courage also is required to sit with patients whose wasted bodies and inability to manage the most intimate functions of daily life have robbed them of those aspects of life on which we rely to maintain our sense of dignity. At the deepest level those who care for dying patients must have resolved for themselves questions that arise from the realization of life's finitude. Only if we face these questions with courage can we offer care with openness and hope.

Hope, the other requirement for being part of God's adventure, assumes a special meaning when a patient faces end-stage care. In the case of AIDS patients, hope can be even more elusive. Often even those resources available to other people—the support of family members and a sense of personal privacy and dignity—are absent or greatly reduced. Hope for the AIDS patient does not at present include the hope of getting well. The prayers of well-

intentioned people for physical healing may seem a mock-
ery. In the face of death, hope takes on other meanings:
hope that what is left of life can be lived with dignity; hope
that one will not die alone; hope that one's suffering will
in some small way contribute to the resolution of the
crisis.

A crucial identifying feature of the community of God's
people is that it remains open to the stranger. To remain
open to the stranger with AIDS, to love this stranger,
requires a special measure of courage and hope which, left
to our own resources, we achieve only partially. In the face
of societal prejudice and hysteria, the willingness to reach
out and touch the life of a man, woman, or child with
AIDS is possible only to grace-filled people empowered by
a Spirit who promises always to counsel and strengthen us.
For such a grace-filled people there can be no disparity
between words and deeds. If the community is to be a
community of integrity, the "doing" of the community
must be an expression of its "being," and that being, both
for the community and for its individual members, is established by God's self-disclosure. And therein lies the
rub. Jesus spoke in terms of finding life only when we are
prepared to lose it in ministry to others. At least we are
warned that this is a "hard saying" and that we should not
attempt to follow Jesus unless we have counted the cost.
Discipleship which issues in loving service to others then
becomes a matter not only of how responsive we are to the
servant-leader who strides ahead toward Jerusalem but of
how responsible we are in manifesting that response in our
ministries. Membership in God's community is not a free
ride; it involves the readiness to lose our lives for Jesus'
sake and for the sake of the gospel. And we should not
imagine this saying to be mere hyperbole.

The scriptures help God's people to understand that we
are called to fill a servant role. The term "servant"—or,
more accurately, "slave"—was accepted by Jesus as the
inner core of his person and mission, and it must become
ours. Paul was not deterred from applying the title to
himself. He gloried in it and urged his fellow servants to

appropriate its meaning for their own lives. Jesus upbraided his friends when they pointedly rejected a servant role on entering the upper room for the Passover meal (Luke 22:24–27). It is only through sharing in Jesus' servanthood that his fellow servants become heirs with him to God's promises (Gal. 3:29; Titus 3:7; Heb. 6:17). Sharing in Jesus' servanthood means sharing in his work, the "work" of loving one another as fellow slaves and joint heirs to God's grace (1 John 4:7–12; see also John 13:34–35). In the Johannine account of the Last Supper, Jesus washed the disciples' feet. His message is explicit: "I have set you an example: you are to do as I have done for you" (John 13:15).

Like other images in the scriptures, the image of prophet derived from the lives of Old Testament figures is rich in meaning for this discussion. The prophets cared deeply about the moral shape of society. The prophets are best understood not when seen as individuals but when seen in the context of organized society and in the performance of important social roles. The prophetic image applied to the church implies that it must either accept the values and derivative decisions of the larger society or, when its own values differ from those of society, stand and confront them. It is doubtful if keeping silent is a response that God will countenance. The prophets did not keep silent. Their presence was a destabilizing force at the king's court, the place where decisions were made.[1] The prophets consistently charged that the system was not to be equated with reality, that alternatives were thinkable, and thus the values and the claims of the system were subject to criticism.

Is there a message here for God's people in the midst of the AIDS crisis? We believe there is. If people are excluded from society, they may in fact be unable to make themselves heard above the clamor of representatives of government—national or local—debating with one another, or the hostile voices of citizens demanding that AIDS patients (including young children) be segregated from the rest of society. Just as the prophets could not remain silent in the face of oppression, the church's voice must be raised in defense of the outcast. For this cause also, Jesus' voice is raised on behalf of people who had been cast out of their communities. In this matter also he has given an example that we are to do for one another what he has done for us.

Not surprisingly, there are drawbacks to adopting the role of prophet. It can be a life-threatening role, as the prophets found. Elijah fled for his life from Queen Jezebel. Her ruthless response to a poor farmer had shown that there are no limits to greed when the system permits oppression. Because Elijah challenged the system, Jezebel vowed to destroy him. The challenge to God's people is that even in the face of dire threat, the establishment must be called into question by God's prophets when civil power is used to isolate and further deprive the helpless and excluded. Only through such action can a way be opened so that God's love can be extended to the outcast. If the church does not speak for the outcast at that moment, the outcast may miss God's invitation to enter into the joy of the kingdom. If the people of God fail to act, Jesus warns his followers, they will be excluded from the kingdom themselves. If speaking for "the poor" places the church in situations of risk, it should come as no surprise (see Mark 8:34–38).

The AIDS crisis is thus a challenge to the church to be in the forefront, filling a servant-leader role, beckoning the larger community to follow, providing adequate resources to people whose lives are blighted by the AIDS virus. Being God's voice is not enough, however. The church is to do God's will by loving and serving the needs of patients and families, whether or not society acts. This obedient response should be an interfaith ministry for several reasons. First, the public response to people with AIDS and their families has been so vitriolic that programs designed to serve them will be received with greater seriousness if developed and endorsed by local religious leaders acting together and speaking to the civic community with one voice. The churches should join hands with the Jewish community and other concerned groups. Such a united effort can stand as an expression of the ability of God's people to undertake joint projects that are redeeming and compassionate, aligning deeds with words. It may be added parenthetically that there is something tragic in the fact that often it takes a crisis to motivate God's people to manifest the unity which God's word indicates is expected of us. The AIDS crisis presents this opportunity. Only if the challenge is accepted can we expect the civil government to assume its own particular responsibility.

Second, the costs to people who respond to the needs of people with AIDS are heavy. The level of nurture and support necessary to sustain such efforts can best be provided by an ecumenical response. An individual rabbi or pastor may be misrepresented and denigrated if he or she expresses concern for people with AIDS. But if neighborhood clergy and laity act together, their voices will be heard more widely and can evoke a more concerted response. Such joint action also provides a stronger and broader basis for community education. In the same manner, if church and synagogue act and speak together at the civic level, their united efforts not only are more likely to receive appropriate attention, they also will be able to address community concerns related to the AIDS crisis with greater effect.

Third, the nature and scope of the epidemic makes AIDS a national concern. While much of the response is local in nature, many aspects of the crisis are best addressed at federal legislative and executive levels. Funding for research, the protection of AIDS patients from exploitation, and access to social welfare resources are issues upon which local action will have little bearing. There is, therefore, a need for nationwide ecumenical action to influence these decisions. At that level, as much as in local communities, religious bodies can exercise more influence if they speak with one voice. At that level also, the representative bodies may project a sense of unity for which there are all too few opportunities.

The problem of how to disseminate information regard-

ing AIDS is one that Jews and Christians could address
with a single national voice. The debate about how to
discuss matters of sex and sexually transmitted diseases—
and especially whether and by what means they ought to
be confronted through public education—continues to be
intense and bitter in the United States. It may well be that
the AIDS epidemic will force disparate groups in society
to arrive at mutually acceptable approaches to the underlying controversies. In any case, the emergence of AIDS
confronts the religious community with the opportunity
to develop study materials for all ages focused on the
nature and meaning of human sexuality and sexual relationship.

There is probably even deeper ignorance and misunderstanding of the factors that contribute to the emergence of
the drug culture and the entrapment of particular individuals within it. Perhaps the time has come to begin to
look for answers to certain nagging questions. Does our
society, as presently constituted, contribute to the very
destructiveness that it publicly condemns? Does the intensity of competition, from which springs an unending drive
to succeed, contribute to the use of either soft or hard
drugs? Can congregations assist people to identify and
explore courses of action that could prevent the very situations which, if unaddressed, may result in antisocial and
self-destructive conduct? It is a fact that the local congregation is one of the most widespread forms of social organization. It suggests itself, at this moment, as a forum in
which these concerns can be explored to the benefit of
members and the community at large. And without in any
way reducing the role of lay members in bringing effective
programs into being, cultural roles place clergy in a
unique position to initiate and support AIDS-related educational and service projects. Thus churches and syna-
gogues may be agents for health and reconciliation in a
society at risk and in need of leadership.

The words that demand attention in the tragic drama
of AIDS are *urgency, challenge, opportunity,* and *task.*
The situation of people with AIDS is one of unprece-

dented and chronic grief, demanding an intense pastoral response from the religious community. AIDS is an unparalleled crisis, not only because it remains incurable but because of the stigma that quickly attaches to the disease, and those it afflicts, and its potential to destroy lives and communities. It is a situation that cries out for a redemptive response, one from which the people of God dare not turn away. There are both immediate and long-term tasks to be performed. The task at hand is to constitute an accepting community, concerned for the needs of patients and others affected by AIDS, and to minister to them. Long-term tasks and challenges relate to the obligation to understand and educate people regarding the complex factors that have contributed to AIDS and the spread of HIV. We urge congregations to develop joint neighborhood projects to ensure that their members and communities are familiar with the relevant medical and psychosocial data. It is our hope that such efforts will result in the development of joint projects of ministry to individuals and families in need of care. The church is confronted with the opportunity to make credible the New Testament image of God's people as a reconciling and redeeming community. If we fail in this endeavor, it will be a failure not only of nerve, but also of love.

Notes

Chapter 1: The AIDS Crisis

1. Dennis Altman, *AIDS in the Mind of America* (Garden City, N.Y.: Doubleday & Co., Anchor Books, 1986), p. 26.

2. Many case reports of people with AIDS or AIDS-related complex and their lovers, families, and clinicians are contained in another book by the authors; see Earl E. Shelp, Ronald H. Sunderland, and Peter W. A. Mansell, *AIDS: Personal Stories in Pastoral Perspective* (New York: Pilgrim Press, 1986).

3. Charles E. Rosenberg, *The Cholera Years: The United States in 1832, 1849, and 1866* (Chicago: University of Chicago Press, 1962), p. 4.

4. Ibid., p. 40.

5. Ibid., pp. 118, 120–121.

6. Ibid., pp. 200–220.

7. Allan M. Brandt, *No Magic Bullet: A Social History of Venereal Disease in the United States Since 1880* (New York: Oxford University Press, 1985).

8. Quoted by Brandt, p. 180.

9. Ibid., p. 5; see Joan Ablon, "Stigmatized Health Conditions," *Social Science and Medicine* 15B (1981),

5–9. Other articles in this issue may also be of interest to the reader.

10. Brandt, pp. 132, 168.

11. Ibid., pp. 23, 157, 168.

12. Ibid., p. 159.

13. Quoted by Brandt, p. 183, from the *New York Times* (June 17, 1983).

14. Altman, p. 16. See also Robert Bazell, "The History of an Epidemic," *New Republic* (August 1, 1983), pp. 14–18.

15. See "The New Untouchables," *Time* 126 (September 23, 1985), 24–26; "The Real Epidemic: Fear and Despair," *Time* 122 (July 4, 1983), 56–58; and "AFRAIDS," *New Republic* 193 (October 14, 1985), 7–10.

16. This incident was widely reported in Houston and across the nation. See "The Backlash Builds Against AIDS," *U.S. News & World Report* 99 (November 4, 1985), 9.

17. Quoted by Jonathan Lieberson, "The Reality of AIDS," *New York Review of Books* (January 16, 1986), p. 46.

18. William F. Buckley, Jr., "Crucial Steps in Combating the AIDS Epidemic," *New York Times* (March 18, 1986), p. 27.

19. John R. Emshwiller, "LaRouche-Supported Initiative on AIDS Policy in California Spurs Debate on Handling Disease," *Wall Street Journal* (August 11, 1986), p. 34.

20. "AIDS Fears of the Unmarried," *New York Times* (January 22, 1986), p. A17.

21. "A Newsweek Poll: Sex Laws," *Newsweek* 108 (July 14, 1986), 38.

22. "The Church's Response to AIDS," *Christianity Today* 29 (November 22, 1985), 50; "Jerry Falwell: Circuit Rider to Controversy," *U.S. News & World Report* 99 (September 2, 1985), 11.

23. Jerry Fallwell, "AIDS: The Judgment of God," *Liberty Report,* April 1987, p. 5.

24. Jerry Fallwell, "How Many Roads to Heaven?" Old Time Gospel Hour-760 (audio tape).
25. Earl E. Shelp and Ronald H. Sunderland, "AIDS and the Church," *Christian Century* (September 11–18, 1985), pp. 797–800.
26. Eileen P. Flynn, *AIDS: A Catholic Call for Compassion* (Kansas City, Mo.: Sheed & Ward, 1985). For a cleverly written, misleading, and sensationalizing examination of AIDS published by a Catholic press that contrasts with Flynn, cf. Gene Antonio, *The AIDS Cover-Up? The Real and Alarming Facts About AIDS* (San Francisco: Ignatius Press, 1986).
27. William E. Swing, "Open Letter to the Reverend Charles Stanley," January 18, 1986, unpublished.
28. John R. Quinn, "The AIDS Crisis: A Pastoral Response," *America* (June 28, 1986), pp. 504–506.
29. John J. O'Connor, "The Archdiocese and AIDS," *Catholic New York* (September 19, 1985), p. 21.
30. "Resolution on Acquired Immune Deficiency Syndrome (AIDS)," Adopted by the Fourteenth General Synod, United Church of Christ, Pittsburgh, Pennsylvania, June 24–28, 1983.
31. Resolution adopted by the 68th General Convention of the Episcopal Church, Anaheim, California, September 7–14, 1985.
32. "Resolution on Ministry in the Midst of the AIDS Epidemic," General Board of Discipleship, United Methodist Church, February 25–28, 1986. The General Board of Global Ministries of the United Methodist Church adopted on April 11, 1986, a statement titled "The Church as a Healing Community and the AIDS Crisis." This statement calls for compassionate ministries, rejects claims that AIDS is punishment, opposes homophobia, and asks that the rights of affected persons be protected.
33. We do not imply by not cataloging representative statements about AIDS by persons and bodies of other denominations that they are less important. We cannot provide a comprehensive list of all such statements, pro and con. Our concern is to call attention to the moderate

and compassionate tone of these resolutions in contrast to statements by conservative columnists and fundamentalist clergy.

34. See Selected References for a sampling of articles describing these ministries.

Chapter 2: The AIDS Epidemic

1. Thousands of medical and scientific articles have appeared in learned journals about the AIDS virus, HIV, its effects on the body, clinical features of the syndrome, treatments, epidemiology, and potential vaccines. Entries in this bibliography are accessible by computer at many libraries. The facts about AIDS presented in this chapter reflect this wealth of data and our experience. Citations, however, are restricted to a few summary references that are generally available (see Selected References). The bibliographies in these materials direct the reader to more technical works.

2. Jean L. Marx, "AIDS Virus Has a New Name—Perhaps," *Science* 232 (May 9, 1986), 699–700; and "Human Immunodeficiency Viruses," ibid., 697.

3. Gallo, "The AIDS Virus," p. 56.

4. Other blood assays that can be used to detect or confirm infection are Western blot, radioimmune assay, and immune fluorescence.

5. Our references to AIDS include adult and pediatric cases. The diagnostic criteria differ for the two populations, however. The CDC definition for adult AIDS is reprinted in Institute of Medicine, *Confronting AIDS*, pp. 316–319. The definition of AIDS for children appeared in Centers for Disease Control, *Morbidity and Mortality Weekly Report* 33 (January 6, 1984), 691.

6. Each of these diseases is described in lay terms in Institute of Medicine, *Mobilizing Against AIDS*, pp. 150–152. A more elaborate classification system for manifestations of HIV infection was issued by the Centers for Disease Control in May 1986. This system includes diseases other than the restricted inclusion criteria for AIDS. As

a consequence, it presents a more comprehensive and accurate picture of diseases related to HIV infection. As such, clinicians find it useful to signal diseases that may warrant further investigation to determine if an underlying HIV infection is responsible. See Centers for Disease Control, *Morbidity and Mortality Weekly Report* 35 (May 23, 1986), 334–339.

7. See Karen J. Chayt et al., "Detection of HTLV-III RNA in Lungs of Patients with AIDS and Pulmonary Involvement," *Journal of the American Medical Association* 256 (November 7, 1986), 2356–2359.

8. See Levy et al., Stoler et al., Gartner et al., and Thomas et al.

9. Ann M. Hardy et al., "The Economic Impact of the First 10,000 Cases of Acquired Immunodeficiency Syndrome in the United States," *Journal of the American Medical Association* 255 (January 10, 1986), 209–211.

10. Ann M. Hardy, "Planning for the Health Care Needs of Patients with AIDS," *Journal of the American Medical Association* 256 (December 12, 1986), 3140. See Anne A. Scitovsky, Mary Cline, and Philip R. Lee, "Medical Care Costs of Patients with AIDS in San Francisco," and George R. Seage III et al., "Medical Care Costs of AIDS in Massachusetts," *Journal of the American Medical Association* 256 (December 12, 1986), 3103–3106 and 3107–3109, respectively.

11. Although public policy and ethical issues related to AIDS have not been addressed extensively, articles and reports are beginning to appear. See Institute of Medicine, *Confronting AIDS,* pp. 95–137; and Purtilo et al.; Mills et al.; Dilley et al.; Steinbrook et al.; and Bayer et al.; also, Levine and Bermel, eds., "AIDS: The Emerging Ethical Dilemmas" and "AIDS: Public Health and Civil Liberties."

Chapter 3: Illness in Christian Perspective

1. For an elaboration of this theme, see *The Pastor as Theologian,* Earl E. Shelp and Ronald H. Sunderland, eds. (New York: Pilgrim Press, in press).

2. Paul S. Minear, *The Gospel According to Mark,* vol.
17 of the Layman's Bible Commentary, Balmer H. Kelly,
ed. (Atlanta: John Knox Press, 1960), p. 109.
   3. Ibid.
   4. This was the case, for example, with respect to leprosy. In this respect, it is important to recognize that the
term to which reference is made in the Jewish scriptures
and in the New Testament carried a different connota-
tion from that of the disease known commonly as leprosy in the twentieth century. The leprosy of the ancient
Near East actually encompassed a range of dermatologi-
cal disorders that seldom approached the seriousness or
evoked the level of fear with which today's leprosy
(Hansen's disease) is associated. Such common skin diseases as psoriasis, eczema, and other common rashes and
lesions were probably included under the general heading of "leprosy."
   The real suffering of lepers was not so much due to
physical discomfort as to the isolation and ostracism that
sufferers met in the general community. It is a similar
isolation and ostracism experienced by people with AIDS
that links the two. More important, given this association,
the response of Jesus to people with leprosy suggests the
model for the response of God's people to people with
AIDS.
   5. T. W. Manson, *The Sayings of Jesus* (London: SCM
Press, 1954), p. 273.
   6. Edward Schillebeeckx, *Jesus: An Experiment in
Christology* (New York: Crossroad Publishing Co., 1985),
p. 184.
   7. Ibid., p. 180.
   8. For a development of the concept that illness and
affliction place the sick person "nearer to death," see
Klaus Seybold and Ulrich B. Mueller, *Sickness and Healing* (Nashville: Abingdon Press, 1981). They state, "The
sick person as such has fallen into death's realm of power,
not only because sickness possibly brings death . . . but
because sickness *eo ipso* belongs to death's domain"
(p. 123).

9. *Nicene and Post-Nicene Fathers,* Series 2, Philip Schaff and Henry Wace, eds., vol. 1, *Eusebius* (Grand Rapids: Wm. B. Eerdmans Publishing Co., 1979), p. 307.

10. John Calvin, *Tracts and Treatises on the Doctrine and Worship of the Church,* vol. 2 (Grand Rapids: Wm. B. Eerdmans Publishing Co., 1958), p. 127.

11. Charles A. Coulson, *Science and Christian Belief* (Chapel Hill, N.C.: University of North Carolina Press, 1955), p. 19.

12. Dorothee Soelle, *Suffering* (Philadelphia: Fortress Press, 1975), p. 22.

13. Ibid., p. 26.

14. John B. Cobb, Jr., and David Ray Griffin, *Process Theology: An Introductory Exposition* (Philadelphia: Westminster Press, 1976), pp. 51–52.

15. The philosopher Alfred North Whitehead suggests that, to the extent that conformity to the divine aims is incomplete, there is evil in the world. New actualities or realities (such as AIDS) may lead not to enjoyment but to discord, a term Whitehead uses to refer to physical or mental suffering which is simply evil in itself, whenever it occurs. See Alfred North Whitehead, *Religion in the Making* (New York: Macmillan Co., 1926), p. 60, and *Adventures of Ideas* (New York: Macmillan Co., 1933), pp. 329–330, 342.

16. See James A. Wharton, "Theology and Ministry in the Hebrew Scriptures," in Earl E. Shelp and Ronald Sunderland, eds., *A Biblical Basis for Ministry* (Philadelphia: Westminster Press, 1981), pp. 62–69.

17. See Alan Keith-Lucas, *Giving and Taking Help* (Chapel Hill, N.C.: University of North Carolina Press, 1972), p. 9.

18. Cobb and Griffin, p. 74.

Chapter 4: God and the Poor

1. R.B.Y. Scott, *The Relevance of the Prophets,* rev. ed. (New York: Macmillan Co., 1969), p. 119.

2. Robert J. Karris, "Poor and Rich: The Lukan *Sitz im Leben,*" in *Perspectives on Luke-Acts,* Charles H. Talbert, ed. (Danville, Va.: Association of Baptist Professors of Religion, 1978), p. 117.

3. Joachim Jeremias, *New Testament Theology: The Proclamation of Jesus* (New York: Charles Scribner's Sons, 1971), pp. 109–113. Jeremias understands the literal use of poor in Luke 6:20 to be the original rather than the religious interpretation given in Matthew 5:3.

Chapter 5: AIDS Ministries

1. For discussions of the mutual influence of religious thought and social life, see Ernst Troeltsch, *The Social Teaching of the Christian Churches,* vol. 1 (New York: Harper & Row, 1960), pp. 23–37; H. Richard Niebuhr, *Christ and Culture* (New York: Harper & Row, Harper Torchbooks, 1956); H. Richard Niebuhr, *The Kingdom of God in America* (New York: Harper & Row, Harper Torchbooks, 1959); Ernest R. Sandeen, ed., *The Bible and Social Reform* (Philadelphia: Fortress Press, 1982); and William A. Clebsch, *From Sacred to Profane America: The Role of Religion in American History* (New York: Harper & Row, 1968).

2. The virtue of courage is examined in theological perspective by Peter Geach, *The Virtues* (Cambridge, Mass.: Cambridge University Press, 1977), pp. 150–170, and by Josef Pieper, *The Four Cardinal Virtues: Prudence, Justice, Fortitude, Temperance* (Notre Dame, Ind.: University of Notre Dame Press, 1966), pp. 115–141. For an analysis of the role of courage in medical contexts, see Earl E. Shelp, "Courage: A Neglected Virtue in the Patient-Physician Relationship," *Social Science and Medicine* 18 (1984), 351–360; and Earl E. Shelp, "Courage and Tragedy in Clinical Medicine," *Journal of Medicine and Philosophy* 8 (November 1983), 417–429.

3. Among the sociological literature on male homosexuality, the following may be helpful to people seeking an understanding of gay lifestyles and culture: Bell and

Weinberg, *Homosexualities;* Tripp, *The Homosexual Matrix;* G. Weinberg, *Society and the Healthy Homosexual;* M. S. Weinberg and C. J. Williams, *Male Homosexuals;* Altman, *Homosexual* and *The Homosexualization of America;* and J. D'Emilio, *Sexual Politics, Sexual Communities.*

4. The literature is extensive providing insight into the contributing factors of drug abuse and the difficulty of altering behavior. See Shiffman and Wills, *Coping and Substance Abuse;* Lidz and Walker, *Heroin, Deviance, and Morality;* Arie Cohen, "A Psychosocial Typology . . ."; George Serban, ed., *Social and Medical Aspects of Drug Abuse;* Bernard Segal, "Intervention and Prevention . . ."; Brunswick and Messeri, "Drugs, Lifestyle, and Health"; and Newcomb and Bentler, "Substance Use and Ethnicity."

5. See chapters 3 and 4.

6. The role of freedom in ministry is expertly analyzed by James A. Wharton in "Theology and Ministry in the Hebrew Scriptures," in Earl E. Shelp and Ronald Sunderland, eds., *A Biblical Basis for Ministry* (Philadelphia: Westminster Press, 1981), pp. 17–71.

7. The National Library of Medicine publishes a bibliography of medical and scientific articles regarding AIDS. The total number of entries from March 1980 through March 1986 exceeds 4,500. This number does not include popular and nonscientific scholarly publications about AIDS. It may be that no other phenomenon in history has been subjected to such an extensive inquiry in so brief a time.

8. The discussion of homosexuality by moral theologians has been active in recent years. Several authors have rejected or questioned biblical and theological condemnations of homosexual people. See George Edwards, *Gay-Lesbian Liberation;* Robert Nugent, ed., *A Challenge to Love;* James Nelson, *Embodiment;* John Boswell, *Christianity, Social Tolerance, and Homosexuality;* Scanzoni and Mollenkott, *Is the Homosexual My Neighbor?;* and Earl Shelp, "Pastor, I Think I'm Gay." A contrary, disapprov-

ing, and unaccepting argument is contained in the Roman Catholic Doctrinal Congregation's Letter to Bishops, "The Pastoral Care of Homosexual Persons," *Origins: NC Documentary Service* 16 (November 13, 1986), 378–382.

9. See literature cited in notes 3 and 4 of this chapter.

10. The following is suggestive of the literature on ministry as a duty of ordained and lay people: Hendrik Kraemer, *Theology of the Laity* (Philadelphia: Westminster Press, 1958); Mark Gibbs and Ralph Morton, *God's Frozen People* (Philadelphia: Westminster Press, 1965); Marie Joseph Congar, *Lay People in the Church* (London: Geoffrey Chapman, 1959); Karl Barth, *Dogmatics* IV/3 (Edinburgh: T. & T. Clark, 1962); Lesslie Newbigin, *The Household of God* (London: SCM Press, 1953); C. W. Brister, *Pastoral Care in the Church* (New York: Harper & Row, 1964); John T. McNeill, *History of the Cure of Souls* (New York: Harper & Brothers, 1951); James Fenhagen, *Mutual Ministry: New Vitality for the Local Church* (New York: Seabury Press, 1977) and *Ministry and Solitude* (New York: Seabury Press, 1981); Edward Schillebeeckx, *Ministry* (New York: Crossroads Publishing Co., 1981); Ronald H. Sunderland, "Lay Pastoral Care," *The Journal of Pastoral Care* (in press).

11. Ronald H. Sunderland, "Sustaining Lay Ministry Through Supervision," *The Christian Ministry* 16 (November 1985), 15–17; Gregg D. Wood, "Hospital-based Lay Pastoral Visitation Program," *Journal of Pastoral Care* 40 (September 9, 1986), 163.

12. Wharton (note 6), p. 69.

13. We recommend teams of twenty people per patient. Visitation can be conducted in pairs once every two weeks, thus utilizing fourteen people. The remaining six are substitutes or can be part of a rotation.

14. Prophetic, servant, and priestly ministry are analyzed in the following books edited by the authors: *The Pastor as Prophet* (New York: Pilgrim Press, 1985), *The Pastor as Servant* (New York: Pilgrim Press, 1986), and *The Pastor as Priest* (New York: Pilgrim Press, 1987).

15. For a general discussion of the religious use of taboo, see Mary Douglas, *Purity and Danger* (London: Routledge & Kegan Paul, 1966), chs. 1, 3, and 7–10.

16. Cf. Gerhard von Rad, *Genesis* (Philadelphia: Westminster Press, 1961). Von Rad suggests that the opening chapters of Genesis are etiologic narratives attempting to provide a theological sanction for human observations of the natural and social orders.

17. Public and private agencies have produced excellent educational material. Readers are directed to the local offices of the American Red Cross to obtain written and video resources. The personal stories of patients, families, lovers, and clinicians are told in pastoral perspective in another volume written by the authors; see Earl E. Shelp, Ronald H. Sunderland, and Peter W. A. Mansell, *AIDS: Personal Stories in Pastoral Perspective* (New York: Pilgrim Press, 1986).

18. See Jim Nieckarz, "Our Fragile Brothers: What We Must Learn from AIDS," *Commonweal* (July 12, 1985), 404–406; James B. Nelson, "Responding to Learning from AIDS," *Christianity and Crisis* (May 19, 1986), 176–181; and Martin S. Weinberg and Colin J. Williams, *Male Homosexuals* (New York: Penguin Books, 1975). An intriguing article by a conservative in *National Review* makes the case that homosexual people are the favorite targets of hostility by conservative ideologues. The logic of these attacks is shown to be flawed and the potential consequences, if the rhetoric is believed and acted upon, are contrary to common notions of decency and law. In short, gay activism and coping responses are held to be a foreseeable response to political persecution. See "John Woolman," "Letter from a Friend: A Conservative Speaks Out for Gay Rights," *National Review* 38 (September 12, 1986), 28–31, 38–39; "Woolman" responds to two articles: see also Joseph Sobran, "The Politics of AIDS," *National Review* 38 (May 23, 1986), 22, 24, 26, 51–52; and William F. Buckley, Jr., "Crucial Steps in Combating the AIDS Epidemic," *New York Times* (March 18, 1986), sec. 1, p. 27.

19. Chapter 3 in this volume is a brief examination of these matters, especially as they bear upon the AIDS crisis.

20. Dennis Altman has analyzed the social, political, and psychological impact of AIDS on American society. See *AIDS in the Mind of America* (Garden City, N.Y.: Doubleday & Co., Anchor Books, 1986).

Chapter 6: Concluding Reflections

1. Walter Brueggemann, "The Prophet as Destabilizing Presence," in Earl E. Shelp and Ronald H. Sunderland, eds., *The Pastor as Prophet* (New York: Pilgrim Press, 1985), p. 49.

Selected References

Chapter 1: The AIDS Crisis

"AIDS Center Run by Archdiocese." *New York Times,* October 28, 1985, p. B3.

"AIDS Crisis Action." *Christian Century,* November 20, 1985, p. 1056.

Berger, Joseph. "Working with AIDS Patients Tests Clerics Nationwide in Difficult Ways." *New York Times,* January 10, 1986, p. 11.

"The Church's Response to AIDS." *Christianity Today,* November 22, 1985, pp. 50–52.

Godges, John. "Religious Groups Meet the San Francisco AIDS Challenge." *Christian Century,* September 10–17, 1986, pp. 771–775.

Goldman, Ari L. "Clerics Offering Support on AIDS." *New York Times,* February 24, 1985, p. 32.

"Help for AIDS Victims." *Christian Century,* February 26, 1986, pp. 201–202.

Rohter, Larry. "Pastor Scolds Parish for Rejecting an AIDS Shelter." *New York Times,* September 2, 1985, pp. 1, 25.

Shelp, Earl E., and Ronald H. Sunderland. "Houston's Clergy Consultation on AIDS: Uniting for a Compassionate Reconciliation." *Christianity and Crisis*, March 2, 1987, pp. 64–66.

Chapter 2: The AIDS Epidemic

Bayer, Ronald, Daniel M. Fox, and David P. Willis, eds. "AIDS: The Public Control of an Epidemic." *Milbank Quarterly*, vol. 64 (Supplement 1, 1986).

Cassens, Brett J. "Social Consequences for the Acquired Immunodeficiency Syndrome." *Annals of Internal Medicine*, vol. 103 (November 1986), pp. 768–771.

Cohen, Mary Ann, and Henry W. Weisman. "A Biopsychosocial Approach to AIDS." *Psychosomatics*, vol. 27 (April 1986), pp. 245–249.

DeVita, Vincent T., Jr., Samuel Hellman, and Steven A. Rosenberg, eds. *AIDS: Etiology, Diagnosis, Treatment, and Prevention.* Philadelphia: J. B. Lippincott Co., 1985.

Dilley, James W., Earl E. Shelp, and Steven L. Batki. "Psychiatric and Ethical Issues in the Care of Patients with AIDS." *Psychosomatics*, vol. 27 (August 1986), pp. 562–566.

Flavin, Daniel K., John E. Franklin, and Richard J. Frances. "The Acquired Immune Deficiency Syndrome (AIDS) and Suicidal Behavior in Alcohol-Dependent Homosexual Men." *American Journal of Psychiatry*, vol. 143 (November 1986), pp. 1440–1442.

Gallo, Robert C. "The AIDS Virus." *Scientific American*, January 1987, pp. 46–56.

———. "The First Human Retrovirus." *Scientific American*, December 1986, pp. 88–98.

Gartner, Suzanne, et al. "Virus Isolation from and Identification of HTLV-III/LAV-Producing Cells in Brain Tissue from a Patient with AIDS." *Journal of the American Medical Association*, vol. 256 (November 7, 1986), pp. 2365–2371.

Holland, Jimmie C., and Susan Tross. "The Psychosocial and Neuropsychiatric Sequelae of the Acquired Immunodeficiency Syndrome and Related Disorders." *An-*

nals of Internal Medicine, vol. 103 (November 1985), pp. 760–764.

Institute of Medicine and National Academy of Sciences. *Confronting AIDS: Directives for Public Health, Health Care, and Research.* Washington, D.C.: National Academy Press, 1986.

————. *Mobilizing Against AIDS: The Unfinished Story of a Virus.* Cambridge, Mass.: Harvard University Press, 1986.

Jaret, Peter. "Our Immune System: The Wars Within." *National Geographic,* vol. 169 (June 1986), pp. 706–734.

Laurence, Jeffrey. "The Immune System in AIDS." *Scientific American,* December 1985, pp. 84–93.

Levine, Carol, and Joyce Bermel, eds. "AIDS: The Emerging Ethical Dilemmas." *Hastings Center Report,* August 1985, Special Supplement.

————."AIDS: Public Health and Civil Liberties." *Hastings Center Report,* December 1986, Special Supplement.

Levy, Robert M., Dale E. Bredesen, and Mark L. Rosenblum. "Review Article: Neurological Manifestations of the Acquired Immunodeficiency Syndrome (AIDS): Experience at UCSF and Review of the Literature." *Journal of Neurosurgery,* vol. 62 (April 1985), pp. 475–493.

Mills, Michael, Constance B. Wofsy, and John Mills. "The Acquired Immunodeficiency Syndrome: Infection Control and Public Health Law." *New England Journal of Medicine,* vol. 314 (April 3, 1986), pp. 931–936.

Morin, Stephen F., Kenneth A. Charles, and Alan K. Malyon. "The Psychosocial Impact of AIDS on Gay Men." *American Psychologist,* vol. 39 (November 1984), pp. 1288–1293.

Nichols, Stuart E. "Psychosocial Reactions of Persons with the Acquired Immunodeficiency Syndrome." *Annals of Internal Medicine,* vol. 103 (November 1985), pp. 765–767.

Purtilo, Ruth, Joseph Sonnabend, and David T. Purtilo. "Confidentiality, Informed Consent, and Untoward Social Consequences in Research on a 'New Killer Disease' (AIDS)." *Clinical Research,* vol. 31 (1983), pp. 462-472.

Quinn, Thomas C., Jonathan M. Mann, James W. Curran, and Peter Piot. "AIDS in Africa: An Epidemiologic Paradigm." *Science,* vol. 234 (November 1986), pp. 955-963.

Steinbrook, Robert, et al. "Ethical Dilemmas in Caring for Patients with the Acquired Immunodeficiency Syndrome." *Annals of Internal Medicine,* vol. 103 (November 1985), pp. 787-790.

Stoler, Mark H., et al. "Human T-Cell Lymphotropic Virus Type III Infection of the Central Nervous System." *Journal of the American Medical Association,* vol. 256 (November 7, 1986), pp. 2360-2364.

Thomas, Christopher S., et al. "HTLV-III and Psychiatric Disturbance." *Lancet,* August 17, 1985, pp. 395-396.

Chapter 5: AIDS Ministries

Altman, Dennis. *Homosexual: Oppression and Liberation.* New York: Avon Books, 1973.

————. *The Homosexualization of America: The Americanization of the Homosexual.* New York: St. Martin's Press, 1982.

Bell, Alan P., and Martin S. Weinberg. *Homosexualities: A Study of Diversities Among Men and Women.* New York: Simon & Schuster, 1978.

Boswell, John. *Christianity, Social Tolerance, and Homosexuality.* Chicago: University of Chicago Press, 1980.

Brunswick, Ann F., and Peter Messeri. "Drugs, Lifestyle, and Health: A Longitudinal Study of Urban Black Youth." *American Journal of Public Health,* vol. 76 (January 1986), pp. 52-57.

Cohen, Arie. "A Psychosocial Typology of Drug Addicts and Implications for Treatment." *International Journal of the Addictions,* vol. 21 (1986), pp. 147-154.

D'Emilio, John. *Sexual Politics, Sexual Communities: The Making of a Homosexual Minority in the United States,*

1940–1970. Chicago: University of Chicago Press, 1983.

Edwards, George R. *Gay-Lesbian Liberation: A Biblical Perspective.* New York: Pilgrim Press, 1984.

Lidz, Charles W., and Andrew L. Walker. *Heroin, Deviance, and Morality.* Beverly Hills, Calif.: Sage Publications, 1980.

Nelson, James B. *Embodiment: An Approach to Sexuality and Christian Theology.* Minneapolis: Augsburg Publishing House, 1978.

Newcomb, Michael D., and P. M. Bentler. "Substance Use and Ethnicity: Differential Impact of Peer and Adult Models." *Journal of Psychology,* vol. 120 (January 1986), pp. 83–95.

Nugent, Robert, ed. *A Challenge to Love: Gay and Lesbian Catholics in the Church.* New York: Crossroad Publishing Co., 1983.

Scanzoni, Letha, and Virginia Ramey Mollenkott. *Is the Homosexual My Neighbor?* San Francisco: Harper & Row, 1978.

Segal, Bernard. "Intervention and Prevention of Drug-Taking Behavior: A Need for Divergent Approaches." *International Journal of the Addictions,* vol. 21 (1986), pp. 165–173.

Serban, George, ed. *Social and Medical Aspects of Drug Abuse.* Jamaica, N.Y.: SP Medical and Scientific Books, 1984.

Shelp, Earl E. "Pastor, I Think I'm Gay." *Christian Ministry,* vol. 10 (March 1979), pp. 18–19.

Shiffman, Saul, and Thomas A. Wills. *Coping and Substance Abuse.* Orlando, Fla.: Academic Press, 1985.

Tripp, C. A. *The Homosexual Matrix.* New York: New American Library, 1976.

Weinberg, George. *Society and the Healthy Homosexual.* Garden City, N.Y.: Doubleday & Co., Anchor Books, 1973.

Weinberg, Martin S., and Colin J. Williams. *Male Homosexuals: Their Problems and Adaptations.* New York: Penguin Books, 1975.

Studies in Illinois Poetry

Edited by John E. Hallwas

Stormline Press
Urbana Illinois
1989

PS
310
.145
S78
1989

International Standard Book Number: 0-935153-13-6

Library of Congress Number: 89-061580

Stormline Press, Inc., a non-profit service organization, publishes works of literary and artistic distinction. The press is particularly interested in those works which accurately and sensitively reflect the cultural life of the American Midwest.

Stormline Press, Inc.
P O Box 593
Urbana Illinois 61801

Manufactured in the United States of America

Publication of this book is made possible in part by a grant from the Illinois Humanities Council and the National Endowment for the Humanities. The sponsors would like to thank the Illinois Humanities Council and the National Endowment for the Humanities for their generous support of this project.

Contents

Introduction

John E. Hallwas
Western Illinois University

ILLINOIS POETS fall into two groups: those who have been significantly influenced by their experience in the state and those who have not. For scholars and readers interested in Illinois, the poets in the first group have far greater importance. After all, they both express Illinois culture and provide insight into the human experience there. They give the state a distinctive poetic tradition.

Of course, any fine poet is a cultural asset, so Illinois is proud to claim figures like William Vaughan Moody and Archibald Mac-Leish – along with others who are less well known – despite the lack of relationship between their poems and life in the Prairie State. In other words, the expression of regional culture should not be, and never has been, the criterion for including poets in the canon of Illinois literature. Too much fine poetry has little or no connection to the place where it was written or where the poet once lived.

On the other hand, the chief value of approaching literature from a state (or regional) perspective resides in the revealing of relationships between individual works and a distinctive cultural experience. This is why certain poets – such as Carl Sandburg, Gwendolyn Brooks, and Dave Etter – will always be of greater interest to Illinois (and midwestern) studies than some others from the state. And this is a matter to keep in mind when reading the articles that follow, all of which relate poets and poems to cultural matters and literary developments in Illinois.

However, the central concern here is not to depict the relationships of many poets to a set of regional values or a common Illinois experience, but to interpret their works and evaluate their achievements. After all, Illinois is a large state with a rich multi-ethnic

I

cultural tradition. It has nurtured poets from very different back-
grounds, living in places as remote from each other as frontier
Springfield and contemporary Chicago.

But it is also important to identify relationships or continuities
among the state's poets, for the making of such connections may
yield insights into the human experience in Illinois and teach us to
read certain poems better. For example, in 1832 America's
foremost poet, William Cullen Bryant, traveled in Illinois, medi-
tated on the landscape, and started writing "The Prairies," which
was completed the following year. It expresses the myth of an
emerging good society, a successful, uncorrupted cultural community, rooted in the soil of a new land, and as such, it is a localization
of the American myth. Of course, the mythic pattern that Bryant
expressed was based on his belief in a fundamental reality about
America, not on evidence that Illinois settlers were particularly
good or capable people. But his poem encouraged people to participate in a communal attempt to found and perpetuate a good
society. That is the function of myth, to make concrete a special
perception which helps to unify the members of a cultural community. The prairie, as a distinctively American landform – and a
midwestern one – symbolizes the myth in Bryant's poem. After all,
the prairies were natural gardens, suggestive of human potential in
the pre-lapsarian Garden.

The prairie also has mythic implications in the poetry of Edgar
Lee Masters, Carl Sandburg, and Vachel Lindsay. In "The Prairie:
Sandridge," for example, Masters meditates on the landscape near
his beloved Petersburg, recalling the wonderful agrarian culture
characterized by "plenty, peace, domestic joy" that he had known
as a youth.[1] The mythic good society is in the past, but the prairie
still symbolizes it for receptive individuals like himself. For
Sandburg, who evokes the myth in "Prairie," the good society is
now, "on the prairie heart," where men and women "are all corn-
huskers together."[2] And for Lindsay, the good society is yet to
come, but the prairie is our assurance that it will come, for the
midwestern soil is sacred ground, the repository of "the soul of the
nation," where the spirits of the pioneers "Rise into the living

hearts of us," as he says in "Sons of the Middle West."[3] His short poem "Lincoln," which was later incorporated into "Litany of the Heroes," explicitly encourages us to respond to the fundamental reality that makes America special and that will ultimately bring the good society: "Would I might rouse the Lincoln in you all,/ That which is gendered in the wilderness/ From lonely prairies. . . ."[4] Lindsay's program for creating the good society is conveyed in his three poems that comprise "The Gospel of Beauty." They localize the American myth on Illinois soil.

The reader of Illinois poetry may also detect a recurring sense of betrayal or failure of the American promise, which is to be expected in a tradition where myth has been prominent. One of the earliest and clearest expressions of that is in the poetry of Eliza Snow, who along with other Mormons was forced from Illinois in 1846. She viewed Nauvoo as a religious version of the good society, which could no longer be sustained in America: "Let us go," she says in a poem by that title, "From a country where justice no longer remains,/ From which virtue is fled – where iniquity reigns."[5] In her perception, the good society at Nauvoo did not become less virtuous, but American culture as a whole did, making it impossible for the community to continue.

A similar mythic view is evident in the poetry of Masters. "New Salem Hill" depicts Lincoln's village as a version of the good society, where virtuous pioneers with "prairie dreams" created "a sylvan democracy," only to have it destroyed by the national betrayal of American ideals that came with "The blood of a merchant's war."[6] That is, he felt that the Civil War could have been avoided, but commercial interests in the North promoted the conflict and ultimately destroyed the mythic "Simple and virile, joyous, brave, and free" America of which New Salem was a clear expression.[7] But unlike Eliza Snow, Masters did not leave America or cease to be interested in it. Instead, he wrote *Spoon River Anthology* (1916) about a prairie town where the good society is substantially degenerated. The failure of the American promise is even more evident in his sequel, *The New Spoon River* (1924).

Likewise, the people of Dave Etter's *Alliance, Illinois* (1978) suffer from a loss of community and pervasive spiritual poverty. Many are lonely and frustrated. There is an apparent lack of shared experience. A few have memories of more meaningful days, but the present is bleak. Porter Knox, for example, recalls "Christmastime on the farm near Noon Prairie," but he dies in a pathetic attempt to recapture that past.[8] And Will Goodenow has a vision of the local depot as it used to be, full of activity and excitement, but awakens to find himself "standing in a new parking lot" – an appropriate image of modern man cut off from his cultural roots.[9] Alliance is the Illinois town as cultural failure, the American village in need of Vachel Lindsay.

Chicago, of course, has been an enormously rich symbol of American social failure, as is evident in prose works like William T. Stead's *If Christ Came to Chicago* (1894), Upton Sinclair's *The Jungle* (1906), and James T. Farrell's *Studs Lonigan* (1935). Poetry too has reflected that perspective. The city of Sandburg's *Chicago Poems* (1916), however vital and productive, is in many ways the opposite of Bryant's good society – a community marked by poverty, injustice, child labor, and homelessness. And the people of Gwendolyn Brooks's Bronzeville do not share in the American promise. Their lives are oriented toward death – as with the pool players who will "Die soon" in the frequently reprinted poem "We Real Cool" – and spiritual death is pervasive in that poor black community.[10] In "The Last Quatrain of the Ballad of Emmet Till," for example, the bereaved mother of a murdered youth experiences "Chaos in windy grays/ through a red prairie" – a fine midwestern metaphor for shattered dreams, hopelessness, desolation.[11]

Nelson Algren's prose poem *Chicago: City on the Make* (1951), which is commonly overlooked by students of both poetry and prose, clearly expresses social failure in mythic terms. The prairie beside the lake attracts hustlers who build the city, but they also corrupt it, and "Hustlertown keeps spreading itself all over the prairie grass" until there are only patches of prairie left "between the shadowed canyons of the loop."[13] The American promise symbolized by the prairie is always there – it is part of the essence of the community – but it is obscured, soiled, betrayed, even as the prairie itself is transmuted into "A rumor of neon flowers, bleeding all night long."[13]

Poetry helps us to see other patterns in the Illinois experience too. The British immigrant who came to Springfield in the early 1830s, and who signed his poems with an H., wrote as a man in transition from one place to another. Psychologically he was still attached to his native England, and he asserted that connection in many poems, but he also wrote to make himself at home in Illinois. His poems are a declaration of roots and a discovery of place – an assessment of himself as an "exile" from his native land and an attempt to find an American voice as "The Sangamo Bard." Although he enjoyed the greater freedom of life in Illinois, he also acknowledged that he had abandoned home for a harsh reality, as poems like "The Western Wilds" and "When Will the Spring Return?" reveal. In one of his most effective poems, entitled "Wolves," he portrays a traveler, a stranger to the West, who loses his way on the winter prairie and is killed by wolves. The poem is symbolic of H's sense of isolation and insecurity as an immigrant in the wilderness, a poet in an uncultured place.

In much the same way, Chicago's Latino poets of our own time are in transition between two cultures. Their poems are also an assertion of roots and a reflection of harsh circumstances, as Marc Zimmerman reveals in his groundbreaking study in this volume. In a sense, they too are poets in the wilderness – a hostile place that is not conducive to the establishment of identity. David Hernandez calls his city "the united states/ of amerikka in/ chicago," and he describes it as a place of "dirt stench/ shit whores" and so on, in a poem called "El Hispano."[14] What connects H. and the Latino poets is the continuing immigration-based cultural pluralism of Illinois. After more than 150 years the state is still a place where people are working out a relationship between their roots and a strange, threatening environment.

Another continuity in Illinois poetry is the state's history. Of course, Lincoln is more than just a historical figure: he is a continuing cultural presence, the mythic Man of the People who embodies the nation's ideals. He has been invoked, praised, and employed as a symbol in many Illinois poems. The most notable one is Lindsay's "Abraham Lincoln Walks at Midnight," which portrays the Great Emanicipator as a kind of genius loci of his native Springfield who is still deeply responsive to the struggles of the Family of Man. Another poem that reflects Lincoln's continuing relationship to us is John Knoepfle's "lincoln tomb, a report," in which the Gutzon Borglum sculpture of Lincoln's head in front of the tomb "tells us who we are . . ./ or should have been/ or who we have to be."[15]

For Masters, Lindsay, and Knoepfle poetry has been the means of communing with the Illinois past, not for its own sake but to help us evaluate and re-direct our lives and our culture. Masters' "Black Hawk," for example, asserts that American greed not only led to the destruction of Indian culture but is leading to the destruction of modern culture too, through abuse of the land that was taken from Black Hawk, who symbolizes all of the displaced Indians. In "The Eagle That Is Forgotten" Lindsay views Governor John Peter Altgeld as a crusader for humanity who inspired others to carry on his efforts – and by implication, should inspire all of us as well. And in Knoepfle's "marquette in winter camp, chicago river, 1675," the great Jesuit explorer displays enormous determination to serve God, despite his suffering. He is a model of purposeful action and strength of will – just what is needed in modern America, where "we don't know/ what to do with our lives," as the poet says in "snowflakes and recorders."[16]

One little-known poet who deserves recognition for having employed the state's history effectively is Baker Brownell. His finest work is "Preludes to 1833," which appeared in *Poetry* magazine 100 years later, in 1933. It is a lengthy poem in which the speaker addresses Father Marquette, Jean Baptiste Point de Sable, and Black Hawk, who represent Illinois before the white man changed it, when the Indians "were content/ under the golden pattern of the day" and "asked no salvation."[17] The prairie wilderness is evoked as a timeless idyllic realm, destroyed by the coming of white men, like Marquette, who did not appreciate it for what it was.

Instead of attuning themselves to the land, they brought "patterned hours and stark routines" that engendered "a massive rage of growing."[18] The poem invites comparison with Knoepfle's short lyric "hill prairie," in which the speaker inquires of a noted Indian, "shickshack old winnebago/ what did you see here," and the intuited response is the pristine beauty of the landscape – "the dream we woke from/ before we were ready."[19]

Like Masters, Sandburg, Lindsay, Etter, and Knoepfle, Brownell views the land as intimately bound up with the culture of Illinois, the Midwest, and the nation. In a prose poem called "Soil," which is reminiscent of the early Sandburg, the speaker says, "I have seen rumbling towns erupt from the soil and raise hills of stone and steel into the sun. Where Chicago growls and gnaws at the great bones of America's work, where Pittsburgh stains the sky, there is hunger and the misery of hope, and the howl and hustle of the soil's work goes on."[20] He asks the pioneers who "kindled the passion of the soil" for insight into the culture they established, but they give no answer. "Soil" is a kind of companion poem to "Preludes to 1833," presenting as it does the post-Indian culture of America with its "rage of growing" and consequent lack of cultural continuity.

Like Sandburg, Brownell recognized that America, especially the Midwest, was oriented toward change, not the preservation of traditions. It is precisely that, of course, which has made a distinctive regional culture difficult to sustain in Illinois and the Midwest, especially in a century marked by so many developments in mass culture. Much has vanished from our collective consciousness since Brownell was writing more than fifty years ago. It is not surprising that Dave Etter's "Land of Lincoln" expresses an enormous sense of loss. "Beyond the boarded up church/ A windmill has a face of broken bones," the speaker says, and the great cultural leaders are gone:

> Lindsay gone. Masters gone. Sandburg gone.
> Abe gone. Darrow gone. Altgeld the Eagle gone.
> Little Giant Douglas gone. Stevenson gone.
> Friends, I got the weary blues.[19]

It would be hard to imagine a better brief portrayal of cultural exhaustion in Illinois – and the consequent lack of vision, direction, and enthusiasm.

But in another sense, Lindsay remains, Masters remains, Sandburg remains, and so do Knoepfle, Etter, and others who are still writing. Their poems remain, and new voices emerge. A good example is Dan Guillory of Decatur, whose work recently appeared in *Benchmark: Anthology of Contemporary Illinois Poetry* (1988) and who is the author of an article in the present volume. In a fine poem called "Lost Gardens" Guillory depicts the persistence of native prairie plants – "everything that grew before the Before/ Of homestead-town-and-section lines" – which spring up unbidden in his own ruined garden.[20] They reveal a lingering continuity with "the Old Prairie" and its mythic promise. And the poet-speaker feels at home in Illinois, despite having roots elsewhere, reminding us of what H. knew 150 years ago, that poetry helps to place us in a meaningful cultural tradition, even as it conveys universal aspects of human life.

Readers who spend time with Illinois poetry will discover other continuities and other insights into the experience of people in the state. They will also discover some remarkably talented poets who are part of a rich and fascinating literary tradition. The present volume is intended to help people do that. *Studies in Illinois Poetry* is a collection of papers that were presented at the Benchmark Conference on Poetry in Illinois, held at the Champaign Public Library on April 7-10, 1988. The event was planned and directed by Ray Bial of Stormline Press. It was the first conference, and this is the first book, devoted to the study of Illinois poetry.

Notes

[1] "The Prairie: Sandridge," *Along the Illinois* (Prairie City, IL: James A. Decker Press, 1942), p. 35.

[2] "Prairie," *The Complete Poems of Carl Sandburg*, rev ed. (New York: Harcourt Brace Jovanovich, 1970), pp. 79, 84.

3 "Sons of the Middle West," *The Poetry of Vachel Lindsay*, Vol. 2, ed. Dennis J. Camp (Peoria, IL: Spoon River Poetry Press, 1985), p. 794.

4 "Lincoln," *General William Booth Enters into Heaven and Other Poems* (New York, Mitchell Kennerly, 1913), p. 63. The poems appears in broadside format in volume two of Camp's *The Poetry of Vachel Lindsay* (Peoria, IL: Spoon River Poetry Press, 1984), p. 63, under the title "To the Young Men of Illinois."

5 "Let Us Go," *Poems, Religious, Historical, and Political*, Vol. 1 (Liverpool: F. D. Richard, 1856), p. 146.

6 "New Salem Hill" *Invisible Landscapes* (New York: Macmillan, 1935), pp. 26, 28, 30.

7 Ibid., p. 28.

8 "Porter Knox: The Christmas Tree," *Alliance, Illinois* (Peoria, IL: Spoon River Poetry Press, 1983), p. 212.

9 "Will Goodenow: The Red Depot," *Alliance, Illinois*, p. 35.

10 "We Real Cool," *Selected Poems* (New York: Harper and Row, 1963), p. 73.

11 "The Last Quatrain of the Ballad of Emmett Till," *Selected Poems*, p. 81.

12 *Chicago: City on the Make* (Garden City, NY: Doubleday, 1951), pp. 59, 91.

13 *Chicago: City on the Make*, p. 91.

14 "El Hispano," *Despertando* (Chicago: privately printed, 1971), p. 52.

15 "lincoln tomb, a report," *Poems from the Sangamon* (Urbana: University of Illinois Press, 1985), p. 64.

16 "snowflakes and recorders," *Poems from the Sangamon*, p. 66.

17 "Preludes to 1833," *Poetry*, 41 (1933), p. 297.

18 "Preludes to 1833," pp. 296, 302.

19 "hill prairie," *Poems from the Sangamon*, p. 20.

20 "Soil," *Poetry*, 22 (1923), p. 61.

21 "Soil," p. 60.

22 "Land of Lincoln," *Selected Poems* (Peoria, IL: Spoon River Poetry Press, 1987), p. 53.

23 "Lost Gardens," *Benchmark: Anthology of Contemporary Illinois Poetry* (Urbana, IL: Stormline Press, 1988), p. 142.

Illinois Poetry before the Chicago Renaissance*

John E. Hallwas
Western Illinois University

ILLINOIS POETRY became nationally important in the second decade of the twentieth century, when Vachel Lindsay, Edgar Lee Masters, and Carl Sandburg began writing distinctive, exciting poems based largely on their experience in the state. They were the main poets of the Chicago Renaissance, and for a time they were very highly regarded and widely read. Their literary reputations have since declined, but they are still commonly viewed as poets of distinction, and in Illinois, as John Knoepfle has said, they have "a symbolic stature that is somehow beyond critical appraisal."[1] In other words, they not only have historical importance in the development of modern poetry, they have continuing cultural significance in their home state (and in America as a whole, to a lesser extent). Their poems are still read and admired.

Earlier Illinois poetry is not. Unfortunately, the Chicago Renaissance tends to diminish the significance of what came before it. After all, nineteenth-century Illinois poetry did not create such an impact. It was seldom very innovative, nor did anyone produce a volume comparable to *Spoon River Anthology* (1915) or *Chicago Poems* (1916). Nevertheless, there were some talented poets writing in the state prior to the Chicago Renaissance, and they created a remarkably varied body of poetry that deserves a modern readership. By and large they were public poets, committed to speaking

---

*This study incorporates some comments made in an earlier, shorter article: "Illinois Poetry: The Lincoln Era," in *Selected Papers in Illinois History 1981*, ed. Bruce D. Cody (Springfield: Illinois State Historical Society, 1982), pp. 15-23.

out on current conditions, whether local or national, and in that sense, they were the legitimate forerunners of Lindsay, Masters, and Sandburg. Those earlier poets seldom explored the self, but they left a vivid record of what they felt compelled to write about. A few of them gained national attention, and together they provided the Prairie State with the finest nineteenth-century poetic tradition in the Midwest.

The most famous writer of "Illinois poetry" during the nineteenth century wasn't an Illinois poet. That is, he did not reside in the state. William Cullen Bryant (1794-1878) was born and raised in Cummington, Massachusetts, and he later edited a newspaper in New York. He was already America's most highly regarded poet before he visited Illinois for the first time in 1832. He came west to see two of his brothers, Arthur and John, who had recently settled in Jacksonville. During his stay, he and John rode on horseback to Springfield and then north along the Illinois River as far as Pekin. That trip provided inspiration for "The Prairies," his famous poem of 1833, which was widely reprinted and quoted in early Illinois newspapers and travel books. During the 1830s, all four of Bryant's brothers, and his widowed mother, moved to Princeton in Bureau County, where the poet visited them in 1841, 1846, and 1851. He also invested in land at that frontier village.[2]

Aside from celebrating the state's most famous topographical characteristic, "The Prairies" views the Illinois wilderness in mythic terms, as an Edenic garden. The version of the poem that first appeared in *The Knickerbocker Magazine* during 1834 and was later widely circulated in western newspapers has an opening that explicitly refers to the landscape as Edenic:

> These are the Gardens of the Desert, these
> For which the speech of England has no name –
> The boundless unshorn fields where lingers yet
> The beauty of the earth ere man had sinned –
> The Prairies.[3]

The poet meditates on the mysterious mound builders – "The dead of other days" – who had inhabited the Mississippi Valley centuries earlier, and at the end of the poem he reflects on the coming settlers, "that advancing multitude/ Which soon shall fill these deserts." Through Bryant's imaginative identification with both groups, the prairies become symbolic of the cultural potential of Illinois. The landscape is not forbidding or antagonistic but inviting and supportive. An idyllic cultural community – the mythic American good society – seems inevitable. No wonder "The Prairies" became a kind of signature poem for the state prior to the Civil War. Bryant's famous lyric was the first significant work to make symbolic use of the prairie landscape and the first Illinois poem to have an impact on the minds of Illinoisans.

Another lyric that reflects the Edenic perspective was also inspired by the poet's first visit to Illinois: "The Hunter of the Prairies." It associates freedom with the prairie landscape and presents the frontiersman as a kind of American Adam, at one with the unspoiled wilderness, the mythic garden in which he roams:

> Here, with my rifle and my steed,
> And her who left the world for me,
> I plant me, where the red deer feed
> In the green desert – and am free.[4]

Although Bryant, as a visitor, was not part of the development of poetry within the state, he has some importance to the state's poetic tradition because "The Prairies" was the first widely read poem about Illinois, and it does assess the state's cultural potential. In fact, "The Prairies" and "The Hunter of the Prairies" together evoke the ideals of happy community and individual freedom against which the later reality of life in the state can be measured. And Bryant's coming-and-writing was a kind of symbolic act, an extension of the American poetic muse to Illinois soil.

The finest poet of early Illinois is also the most obscure. His identity is uncertain because he simply signed his lyrics with an H., but there is some evidence that his name may have been John Hancock.[5] Between 1831 and 1846 he published seventy poems in Springfield's *Sangamo Journal* that constitute the most significant poetic achievement of the pre-Civil War Midwest. A footnote to one of the lyrics indicated that it was first published in the London *Literary Gazette*. This led to the discovery of twenty-three additional poems in that journal, which brought the established canon up to ninety-three items. These are probably not all that the poet ever wrote or published, but they are probably all that will ever be discovered.

Because his name has not been identified with any certainty, very little is known about the poet. His poems indicate that he was raised in Cornwall and that he lived in or near London as a young man. He had some kind of association with the Inns of Court, London's famous legal societies. That he received a good education can be deduced from his references to a broad spectrum of authors, from Homer to Byron, as well as his acquaintance with Hindu scripture, classical and Norse mythology, and Arthurian legend. He also knew Latin, French, and Italian, and he had traveled to Spain and Italy before moving to America. H. does not mention when he immigrated to the United States, but he had traveled in eastern North America and Canada before coming to Springfield. Since his first surviving poem in the *Sangamo Journal* appeared in the fall of 1831, he probably had come to that frontier village of about 1,000 people just a few years before. He evidently left Springfield in the mid-1830s and thereafter simply mailed poems to the newspaper, although he did return at least once for a visit, in 1845.

Of course, little is known about the poet's life in Springfield, but he did mention that he was the taverner at Jabez Capp's Grocery (general store and bar). He was a single man who liked to take solitary walks in the countryside but who, nevertheless, enjoyed people and regarded himself as the foremost rhymester in the Springfield area. He liked to refer to himself as "The Sangamo Bard" (the poet of Sangamon County).

Perhaps the most interesting of his *Sangamo Journal* poems are the nine satires which were published between December of 1831 and June of 1833. Six of them are over 100 lines long and a couple run to more than 200 lines. The first to appear, "Hame's the Best

Place After A'," is a comical-satirical narrative that shows the
influence of Robert Burns, especially in the poet's use of Scots
dialect. Related to the New England tall tale tradition, it describes
a visit by the devil to Sangamon County, where he finds the winter
weather harder to put up with than the heat of hell. Another
entertaining poem is "Cauld Comfort," an anti-temperance satire
in which the poet attacks both the logic and the inhumanity of
Springfield's anti-liquor crusaders. Other satires, such as "To the
Small-Beer Poets" and "The Remonstrance," deal with women,
bachelors, marriage, and other love-related matters, sometimes
satirically and sometimes with genuine appreciation.

As the title of "To the Small-Beer Poets" suggests, H. liked to
ridicule the other local poets in print. But in a fine poem called
"Bards and Reviewers" he defends his, and their, commitment to
writing poetry in and about the western frontier. As he points out
in a particularly interesting passage, even minor poets have a
useful function:

> Shakespeares, indeed, they may not be,
> But still, they're poets in degree.
> Milton's vast stores they don't possess,
> And yet, they may not please the less;
> Nor do pretend within their scope
> The ease and elegance of Pope.
> Is there in verse no medium found,
> But all must still be classic ground,
> Sublime, most elegant, profound?
> There are, besides the *dii majores*,
> Or greater gods, the *dii minores* –
> The lesser bards, as we may say,
> Who deal but in the retail way.
> We cannot all be Jabez Capps,
> But stlll may sell good wine perhaps.[6]

Aside from his lively satires, H.'s achievement also includes
romantic nature poetry, such as "Lines on the Approach of
Winter" (which is similar to Whittier's "Snow-Bound") and "To
the Frogs" (which resembles Bryant's "The Prairies"). One of his

best lyrics of nature description is "The Approach of Spring," which refers to some aspects of the season that would have been considered unpoetic by most people of the earlier nineteenth century:

> The mud is everywhere, and in the sty
> The sows and all the little ones are spry.
> Now in the town the dapper clerk appears,
> Early to rise, with quill behind his ear –
> The loafers all are out the sun to meet,
> And politicians buzz in every street.
> Sweet faces now are seen along the way;
> The beaus are smart, and hens begin to lay.[7]

On the other hand, some of the poet's nature lyrics display his recognition that the natural world in the West could be an inhospitable and even dangerous place. Among them is "Wolves," a powerful blank verse study of a winter traveler doomed to die in the snow-covered wasteland of the prairie:

> . . . down he sinks at last, and black despair
> Brings hideous shapes and fancies to his eyes.
> Meanwhile, faintly at first, and mingled with the blast,
> The long, loud howl of wolves upon his track
> Is now distinctly heard.[8]

This poem challenges the prevailing romantic conception of a benign natural world, and it symbolizes the poet's sense of isolation and insecurity as a stranger to the West, an immigrant in the wilderness.

H. also wrote many short philosophical lyrics, most of which are sonnets. "Written Near Springfield Churchyard," for example, is an effective poem that displays his debt to the Graveyard Poets of the late eighteenth and early nineteenth centuries. An even better sonnet on death is "Spirits," which reveals the poet's anxiety about what lies beyond the grave:

> They say, at certain times, without control,
> The buried dead at this dark watch appear;
> A sudden horror tells their presence near,

With shrieks upon the gale that chill the soul.
Such was the sound which late the night winds bore,
Like some poor wretch thrown bleeding on the shore.[9]

H. also wrote two poems with medieval European content. "Taur Arthur" is a meditation on a rock along the coast of Cornwall not far from where he was reared. He celebrates the heritage of Cornwall, and his own heritage as a poet, through the use of Arthurian folklore from that area. "The Hall of Odin" focuses on comradeship and conflict in Valhalla (the Norse heaven) as it examines the role of poetry in medieval Scandanavian culture. There is nothing else quite like it in American poetry.

H. has much in common with the finest Eastern poets of his era, although the best works by Bryant, Whittier, Longfellow, and Lowell are superior to his. Like them, he used conventional poetic forms and easily comprehensible language, he usually wrote on common themes, he was often not probing or subtle enough to be thought-provoking, and his poems lack originality of technique and metaphoric complexity. But his satires contain some of the most vigorous and imaginative poetry yet to appear in America, his best nature poems exhibit vitality of expression, his sonnets powerfully convey his realizations about life and death, and "Taur Arthur" and "The Hall of Odin" are successful poems based on legend and mythology. H. was both a public poet and a personal one, commenting on local matters or cultural concerns in some poems and examining his own situation in others. His achievement alone lends unusual interest to early Illinois poetry. He was the finest poet who lived in the pre-Civil War Midwest.

The most tragic of the early Illinois poets was Robert Goudy, Jr. (1816-1842). Born in Pennsylvania, he moved with his family to Vandalia in 1832 and then to Jacksonville a year or so later. His father launched an early newspaper and established a printshop and book bindery. Goudy began to write poetry while enrolled at Illinois College. After graduating in 1839, he studied medicine at Indianapolis and then returned to Illinois in 1841. He settled at St.

Marys, a hamlet in Hancock County, where he died of congestive
fever the following year. He was only twenty-six. His bereaved
relatives published *The Poetical Remains of Dr. Robert Goudy*
(1842), which is among the earliest collections of poetry to appear
in Illinois.[10]

One of his better poems is a "New Year's Address" that appeared
in the *Jacksonville Illinoian* during January of 1840. At that time,
and for decades afterward, it was traditional for newspapers to
print a poem that chronicled events of the past year in the first
issue of the new year. But Goudy employed that tradition for
satire. Among other things, he mentions that land speculation
"Has well nigh crazied all the nation," and he criticizes President
Martin Van Buren for being slow to deal with America's depressed
economy:

> "Hard times," is still the woeful cry,
> "Derangement in the currency!"
> "Business is dull, the banks suspended,
> All confidence and credit ended" –
> "When will this state of things be mended?"
> . . . .
> The unfortunate body politic
> Has been most dangerously sick.
> And yet the footstep followers say
> These hard times soon will pass away,
> That though the times be rather tight,
> All will directly be set right,
> Whene'er our little sovereign chief
> Shall condescend to give relief.[11]

Goudy's best poem, "To My Pet Toad," which appeared in the
Jacksonville Illinoian during January of 1838, is a burlesque of the
conventional love poetry of that time. Instead of idealizing his
beloved, Goudy praises his "dearest toad," using similar exaggera-
tion:

> The lover sings his fair one's charms,
> Her white and matchless-shapen arms,
> Her graceful form and winning air,

Her ruby lips and auburn hair,
Her rosy cheeks and pretty nose,
Her hands, her feet, and e'en her toes –
But nobler strains my musings task,
More winning charms my sonnets ask.
Thy steps are majesty and grace;
Intelligence beams in thy face;
Each virtue finds within thy breast
A place where it may safely rest;
How fine thy nose, how bright thine eyes,
How red thy tongue – the death of flies![12]

"To My Pet Toad" is an amusing satirical poem. Had Goudy lived longer he might have left a more worthwhile poetic achievement, for at least he clearly recognized the shortcomings of much pre-Civil War poetry. And as the "New Year's Address" and "To My Pet Toad" illustrate, comic and satirical poetry from the nineteenth century is often more successful, more readable than serious poetry simply because writers of humorous verse necessarily avoided the elevated style and conventional language which they felt bound to use in serious poems.

Another forgotten poet, but one more likely to be known by his contemporaries, was Thomas Gregg (1808-1892). Raised on the Ohio frontier, he became editor of a magazine, *The Literary Cabinet and Western Olive Branch*, in St. Clairsville and then lived briefly in Cincinnati before immigrating to Hancock County, Illinois. Determined to promote cultural development in the West, he founded several short-lived newspapers and magazines. He also wrote a history of Hancock County and a biography of Joseph Smith. Although he published no volume of poems, his magazine verse impressed William T. Coggeshall, who reprinted a few of his lyrics in a widely circulated anthology, *Poets and Poetry of the West* (1860).[13]

One of Gregg's most successful lyrics is "December," written late in 1847 while he was a newspaper editor in Warsaw and published in the *Warsaw Signal* on April 8, 1848:

Hoary, frosty, drear December!
  Bleakest of the winter months!
Very well do I remember
  How I loved to greet thee once.
In my boyhood's happy hours –
  In my days of youthful prime –
Then I loved thy sweeping tempests –
  Then I loved the winter time.

Now that I am growing older,
  And the frosts of years appear,
The current of my blood runs colder –
  Thy snows becoming still more drear.
Let me escape thy chilling presence,
  Dreariest of the dreary months,
I cannot greet thee as of yore,
  Or love thee as I loved thee once.[14]

The poem presents an effective contrast between the perspectives of youth and age. In the process, it creates an implied comparison between the late fall of the year and the later years of the speaker's life. Indeed, the lyric clearly suggests that the speaker cannot face the final month of the year with love and gladness any more because it reminds him that he, like the year, is approaching his end. December has become symbolic of death.

Another of Gregg's poems that is still readable and interesting is simply entitled "No!" It was written when the Civil War was dragging on and he, like so many others, was impatient for the Union Army to achieve its purpose. Hence, it criticizes the government's management of the war effort, as in these lines:

No policy in the conduct of the war –
No purpose but the Touch-'em-easy sort –
No cheering news of progress, near or far –
No fighting rebels but for fun and sport –
No tools for faithful allies' hands –
No "shooting sticks" for idle "contrabands" –
No thing for 600,000 men to do,

But in the trenches lie,
And in the trenches die![15]

Lines five and six refer to the issue of arming former slaves. Gregg was in favor of that as a measure which would shorten the war. Because it expresses the sense of frustration and anger that many Northerners felt at that time, the poem is more interesting than most midwestern lyrics of the Civil War period. Had Gregg focused more often on either his frontier experience or the events of his era, he might have left a much more worthwhile body of poetry than he did.

One of the most interesting poetic achievements of the early Midwest was produced by Eliza R. Snow (1804-1887), a Mormon who joined that Church in Ohio, suffered through the troubles in Missouri, and wrote many lyrics while at Nauvoo. Like Goudy and Gregg, then, she lived for a time in Hancock County, which would also produce the state's first noted poet, John Hay. Snow was one of the plural wives of Joseph Smith and, later, of Brigham Young. She eventually became the most influential woman in the church at Salt Lake City. Her finest lyrics focus on the Mormon experience in Missouri and Illinois. They are included in her two-volume collection, *Poems, Religious, Historical, and Political* (vol. I, 1856; vol. II. 1877).[16]

Snow had written poems since her teenage years in Ohio, but the turbulent events in Missouri during the later 1830s launched the most significant period of her poetic career. She became a lyrical commentator on the struggles of the Mormons in the Midwest. The opening lines of "The Gathering of the Saints" proclaim her awakening to that new public role:

Awake! my slumbering Minstrel: thou has lain
Like one that's number'd with the'unheeded slain!
Unlock thy music – let thy numbers flow
Like torrents bursting from the melting snow.[17]

"The Gathering of the Saints" might be termed a brief epic about the Mormons' migration to Missouri and their subsequent

persecution by local mobs. It displays the author's detailed knowledge of the Mormon situation, as in this passage about their
struggle at Adam-ondi-Ahman:

> Hemm'd in by foes – depriv'd the use of mill,
> Necessity inspired their patient skill.
> Tin pails and stove-pipes, from their service torn,
> Are chang'd to graters to prepare the corn,
> That nature's wants may barely be supplied
> They ask no treat, no luxury beside;
> Determin'd to maintain the sacred post,
> In spite of earth, in spite of Satan's host![18]

As one might expect, the poem fails to probe the causes of the
conflict. Instead, it simply celebrates the Saints and condemns
their enemies.

Among her poems about the Mormons' difficulties in Illinois is
"The Assassination of Generals Joseph and Hyrum Smith," which
presents the magnitude of that act from the Mormon point of view:

> . . . never since the Son of God was slain
> Has blood so noble flowed from human vein
> As that which now on God for vengeance calls
> From "freedom's" ground – from Carthage prison walls!
> . . . .
> Oh wretched murd-rers! fierce for human blood!
> You've slain the prophets of the living God,
> Who've borne oppression from their early youth
> To plant on earth the principles of truth.[19]

Other interesting lyrics by Snow include "Let Us Go," which
captures the mood of church members after the murders, and
"Camp of Israel No. 2," which describes the beginning of the now-
famous Mormon trek to the Great Salt Lake Valley in 1846.

Although not profound or structurally complex, Eliza Snow's
best lyrics are strikingly original in subject matter, rhythmically
powerful, and remarkably free from the all-too-common excesses
of romantic diction and sentimentality. Unlike so many other poets
of early Illinois, she was able to reflect the reality of her

experience on the frontier. And she was the only woman in the state during the nineteenth century who wrote lyrics of continuing interest – at least to those who study the development of midwestern poetry.

A more talented figure is John Howard Bryant (1807-1902), the youngest brother of America's most famous pre-Civil War poet, William Cullen Bryant. Like his older brother, John was raised in the Berkshires, but he immigrated to Illinois in 1831, residing briefly in Jacksonville before spending the rest of his long life in Princeton. His poetic output was meager, perhaps because he was busy with so many other concerns. Aside from being a pioneer farmer, he was extensively involved in government and politics, was a newspaper editor for a time, and was active in a variety of community and state affairs. As an Illinois legislator, he knew Abraham Lincoln; as an abolitionist, he was an associate of Owen Lovejoy. His literary canon is limited to a single collection, which was twice expanded and published under a different title: *Poems* (1855), *Poems Written from Youth to Old Age* (1885), and *Life and Poems of John Howard Bryant* (1894).[20]

Bryant wrote a number of poems that were based on the Illinois landscape around Princeton, but there is little sense of a unique locale in them. Rather, he chose to focus on his own emotional response to the natural world. Greatly influenced by his famous brother, Bryant wrote primarily meditative nature lyrics and sonnets. His favorite theme is transience, which is also common in his brother's poetry.

Among his pre-Civil War lyrics is "Temperance," which was "Read before the Princeton (Ill.) Washingtonian Society" in December of 1840. It is Bryant's only poem on this exceedingly common topic in early midwestern poetry, and it is one of his finest achievements. He views the controversial matter within the Christian temporal framework, extending from Eden to the Millennium, in order to assert the importance of temperance to man's physical and spiritual well being. In the process, he associates alcohol with temporality and sorrow, water with eternity and joy,

and then concludes that temperance will undo the effects of the
Fall:

> Then let us all our steps retrace,
> Regenerate our wasted race;
> Temperance shall lengthen out the span
> Allotted here on earth to man,
> Bring in the coming years to view,
> The reverent age the patriarchs knew,
> Give to the glad Millennium birth,
> And make a paradise on earth.[21]

Although not a brilliant poem, "Temperance" displays Bryant's
fine sense of structure and his ability to use poetry to analyze his
subject matter.

Sonnets are also an important part of his achievement. One of
his best is simply entitled "Sonnet," and it describes a frontier
preacher at work. Bryant's gift for creating effective rhythms is
especially evident in this lyric:

> I saw a preacher in the house of God;
> With frantic gestures and in accents loud
> And words profane he spread his hands abroad
> And poured anathemas upon the crowd.
> His speech was set with many a phrase uncouth,
> And frivolous remark and common jest;
> A mixture strange of folly and of truth,
> With fierce denunciations for the rest.
> Is this, I thought while listening to his strains,
> A follower of the meek and lowly one?
> Are these the accents heard on Bethleh'm's plains
> When angels hailed the birth of Mary's Son?
> Is this the Gospel sent us from above
> Whose words are peace and charity and love?[12]

The poem is a thought-provoking criticism of the hellfire-and-
histrionics style of preaching that Peter Cartwright and others
practiced in early Illinois. Undoubtedly, Bryant reacted negatively
to the preacher because he himself was a member of the Congregational Church, whose ministers did not indulge in the emotional-

ism that was so characteristic of the Methodists, Campbellites, and other frontier sects.

Bryant's antislavery sympathies are evident in some or his best poems, which also reveal that he viewed himself as a public poet, employing his poetic talent to comment on American culture. In an 1858 lyric called "Hymn," for example, he speaks as the conscience of America, expressing his desire for the freedom of the slaves:

> Upon the nation's heart
>   A mighty burden lies;
> Two hundred years of crime and tears,
>   Of anguish, groans, and sighs.
>
> How long, O Lord! how long!
>   Crushed, trampled, peeled, and dumb,
> Shall thy bound children suffer wrong,
>   And no deliverer come?[23]

Of course, prior to 1860, Bryant probably did not suspect that the deliverer might be Lincoln, his friend from the Illinois legislature. But when the emancipation finally took place, and the assassination closely followed, the poet could not help but view his fellow Illinoisan as a martyr for freedom, which is his perspective in a fine sonnet called "Death of Lincoln":

> "Make way for Liberty," cried Winkelried,
> And gathered to his breast the Austrian spears.
> Fired with fresh valor at the glorious deed,
> O'er the dead hero rushed those mountaineers
> To victory and freedom. Even so
> Our dear, good Lincoln fell in freedom's cause.
> And while our hearts are pierced with keenest woe,
> Lo, the black night of slavery withdraws,
> And liberty's bright dawn breaks o'er the land.
> Four million bondmen, held in helpless thrall,
> Loosed by his word, in nature's manhood stand,
> And the sweet sun of peace shines over all.
> The blood that stained the martyr's simple robe
> Woke the deep sympathies of half the globe.[24]

Through the comparison to Winkelried, the Swiss hero of the fourteenth century, Bryant conveys the notion that Lincoln is just as much a martyr as one who died in battle. But unlike Winkelried's sacrifice, which had a comparatively limited effect, Lincoln's death "Woke the deep sympathies of half the globe." Moreover, this reference to awakening in the final line is prepared for by the dawn imagery that conveys the impact of the emancipation in lines eight and nine. In other words, Bryant sees the emancipation and the assassination as part of the same historical event, bringing the dawn of a new era of liberty in the world.

Almost twenty years later, he wrote another lyric called "At the Tomb of Lincoln," which he read at the dedication of the Lincoln monument in Springfield, on April 15, 1884. In that lengthy poem he views Lincoln as the mythic Great Emancipator, the Savior of the Republic, who deserves the perpetual appreciation and veneration of the American people:

> Not one of all earth's wise and good
>   Hath earned a purer gratitude
> Than the great soul whose hallowed dust
>   This structure holds in sacred trust.
>
> How fierce the strife that rent the land
>   When he was summoned to command!
> With what wise care he led us through
>   The fearful storms that round him blew!
>
> Calm, patient, hopeful, undismayed,
>   He met the angry hosts arrayed
> For bloody war, and overcame
>   Their haughty power in freedom's name.
>
> Mid taunts and doubts the bondman's chain
>   With gentle force he cleft in twain,
> And raised four million slaves to be
>   The chartered sons of liberty.[25]

Bryant was the first Illinois poet of any talent to celebrate Lincoln, and his mythic perspective was shared by many later writers of poetry and prose, including Carl Sandburg and Vachel

Lindsay. He continued to write poems until the end of the century, leaving a small but significant canon behind when he died at the age of ninety-five. His best poems, such as "Temperance," "Hymn," and "Death of Lincoln," are among the most notable achievements of early midwestern poetry.

After the Civil War, some Illinois poets became nationally known. The first and most distinctive of those was John Hay (1838-1905). Born in Salem, Indiana, he was brought to Warsaw, Illinois, three years later. His father, Charles Hay, was a frontier physician with literary interests, and he taught his son Latin and Greek. Young Hay was sent to a private school in Pittsfield from 1849 to 1852, and then he attended Illinois State University (now Concordia College) in Springfield. He received a master's degree from Brown University in 1858, at the age of nineteen. After the election of 1860, President Lincoln appointed Hay as one of his private secretaries. Following the assassination, Hay served as a diplomat in Paris, Vienna, and Madrid, and then he was Assistant Secretary of State under President Hayes. During the post-Civil War period, he became acquainted with such noted American authors as Henry Adams, Bret Harte, Henry James, and Mark Twain. Hay later served as Ambassador to England and then as Secretary of State under presidents McKinley and Roosevelt. He has a significant place in American diplomatic history.[26]

Hay also pursued a literary career after the Civil War. He drew upon his Illinois frontier background for a group of dialect poems called Pike County Ballads that appeared in the early 1870s and gave him a national reputation. He also wrote one novel, *The Breadwinners* (1884), a volume of essays called *Castilian Days* (1871), and a monumental ten-volume life of Lincoln (with John G. Nicolay), which first appeared serially in the 1880s.[27]

Hay wrote many lyrics on common literary topics, but his importance as a poet is based entirely on his Pike County Ballads. At a time when almost all American poetry was characterized by conventional subject matter and stilted formality, Hay's local color realism was lively and original. The opening of "Jim Bludso of the

Prairie Belle," his most famous poem, captures the flavor of oral storytelling as the narrator responds to an apparent inquiry:

> Wall, no! I can't tell whar he lives,
>   Because he don't live, you see;
> Leastways, he's got out of the habit
>   Of livin' like you and me.
> Whar have you been for the last three year
>   That you haven't heard folks tell
> How Jimmy Bludso passed in his checks
>   The night of the Prairie Belle?[28]

"Jim Bludso" is a serious poem that celebrates a rough, irreligious steamboat engineer who dies while saving others during a fire, but most of Hay's Pike County Ballads are humorous. The most famous of those is "Little Breeches," in which a simple-minded speaker narrates the event that prompted his faith in "God and the angels": the survival of his four-year-old son, who was lost in a snowstorm. The poem combines all the elements that made local color writing popular in the period following the Civil War: humor, pathos, dialect, and regionalism.

Both "Jim Bludso" and "Little Breeches" became known throughout the country, and Hay soon wrote other dialect poems, including "Banty Tim," a dramatic monologue which achieves its humorous effect through the speaker's colorful language. Sergeant Tilmon Joy has brought a black soldier (Tim) home with him from the Civil War and, as a result, has run afoul of "the White Man's Committee of Spunky Point," to whom he responds with contempt:

> I reckon I git your drift, gents, –
>   You 'low the boy sha'n't stay;
> This is a white man's country;
>   You're Dimocrats, you say;
> And whereas, and seein', and wherefore,
>   The times bein' all out o' j'int,
> The nigger has got to mosey
>   From the limits o' Spunky P'int!

Le's reason the thing a minute:
   I'm an old-fashioned Dimocrat too,
Though I laid my politics out o' the way
   For to keep till the war was through.
But I come back here, allowin'
   To vote as I used to do,
Though it gravels me like the devil to train
   Along o' sich fools as you.

Now dog my cats ef I kin see,
   In all the light of the day,
What you've got to do with the question
   Ef Tim shall go or stay.
And furder than that I give notice,
   Ef one of you tetches the boy,
He kin check his trunks to a warmer clime
   Than he'll find in Illanoy.[30]

Hay's ability to capture the speech rhythms of the uneducated westerner is clearly evident in these opening stanzas. "Banty Tim" is not only one of the best Pike County Ballads, it is one of the most original and interesting poems related to the Civil War.

Unfortunately, Hay was deeply affected by critics who asserted that his Ballads were simply crude, irreligious doggerel, so he stopped writing them. One, entitled "Benoni Dunn," was not even published until after his death. But the seven dialect poems are clearly his finest achievements. They express his ambivalence toward the frontier, as a place of cultural shallowness and firm values, foolishness and heroism. And they are still entertaining.

Although Asbury Kenyon (1817-1862) and Benjamin Franklin Taylor (1819-1887) were writing in Chicago before the Civil War and were admired locally, they produced no poetry that still deserves to be read. The same is true of Harriet Monroe (1860-1936), who started writing poetry in the 1880s and read her ponderous "Columbian Ode" at the opening of the Chicago World's Fair in 1893. Her only significant work is an autobiography, *A Poet's Life*

(1938), which is notable for its depiction of the Chicago literary scene and the early years of *Poetry* magazine.

The first Chicago poet of any significance was Eugene Field (1850-1895), who came to national attention in the 1880s. He was born in St. Louis and raised there and in Amherst, Massachusetts. After his father's death in 1869, he was sent to study at Knox College in Galesburg. Two years later, he enrolled at the University of Missouri, where he graduated in 1871. He was a reporter and editor for newspapers in St. Louis, Kansas City, and Denver before Melville Stone hired him to write editorials for the *Chicago Daily News* in 1883. Field was an instant success. His "Sharps and Flats" column presented humorous and sentimental verse as well as quaintly humorous and satirical prose, and he became the foremost celebrity in the city. His poems were often reprinted in other newspapers.[31]

Unfortunately, he did not focus on life in Chicago, although one of his lyrics, "Her Fairy Feet," derives its humorous impact from the significance of Chicago as the epitome of harsh, uncultured, modern society:

> "Bring me a tiny mouse's skin,"
>   The boisterous tanner cried;
> "It must be as a rose-leaf thin
>   And scarce three fingers wide."
>
> He seized the fragile, tiny bit
>   Within his brawny hand,
> And cast it in the seething pit,
>   And so the skin was tann'd.
>
> Then came a cobbler to his side,
>   With tools that cobblers use,
> And deft they wrought that mouse's hide
>   Into a pair of shoes.
>
> "Tell me," I asked, "O cobbler, tell
>   For whom these morceaux be?"
> "A lover bade me build them well
>   For his true love," quoth he.

"Where dwells this maid with fairy feet?"
In wonderment I cried;
The old man shifted in his seat –
"Chicago," he replied.[32]

The reversal of expectations was Field's most effective humorous technique, and he also used it in such poems as "One Day I Got a Missive" and "Human Nature," which are among his better works.

A variation of that technique is employed in "The Bibliomaniac's Prayer," in which the speaker, a hopeless devotee of rare books, starts to ask God for the strength to avoid temptation but ends up pleading for a bargain:

Keep me, I pray, in wisdom's way
    That I may truths eternal seek;
I need protecting care today, –
    My purse is light, my flesh is weak.
So banish from my erring heart
    All baleful appetites and hints
Of Satan's fascinating art,
    Of first editions, and of prints.
. . . .
But if, O Lord, it pleaseth Thee
    To keep me in temptation's way,
I humbly ask that I may be
    Most notably beset today;
Let my temptation be a book,
    Which I shall purchase, hold, and keep,
Whereon when other men shall look,
    They'll wail to know I got it cheap.[33]

In this poem Field was speaking from experience, for he was an avid book collector. One of his prose volumes is entitled *Love Affairs of a Bibliomaniac* (1896).

Some of Field's poems are still fun to read, but most of them seem dated and do not appeal to modern readers. A case in point is "Little Boy Blue," a sentimental lyric about the death of a child, which was immensely popular in his own time. Field achieved a certain poignance by focusing on two of the dead child's favorite toys, which are stlll awaiting his return:

> The little toy dog is covered with dust,
>   But sturdy and staunch he stands;
> And the little toy soldier is red with rust,
>   And his musket moulds in his hands.
> Time was when the little toy dog was new,
>   And the soldier was passing fair;
> And that was the time when our Little Boy Blue
>   Kissed them and put them there.[34]

Toward the end of his short life, Field published various collections of his verse and prose, including *A Little Book of Western Verse* (1889) and *With Trumpet and Drum* (1892). Among his books are volumes of lullabies and other poems for children, which made him nationally famous as "the Children's laureate." When he died of heart failure in 1895, at the peak of his career, Chicagoans were shocked and deeply saddened. For a generation or so after his death, his poems for children were widely read in schoolrooms across the country, but his other works were soon forgotten. In truth, he was a poet of little talent, whose significance is largely historical. It is perhaps ironic that this gentle humorist and lullaby collector should be the first notable Chicago poet, but he was.

Richard Hovey (1864-1900) is the only pre-Chicago Renaissance poet of any significance who was born in Illinois, but that is his only connection with the state. Nevertheless, he is commonly viewed as an Illinois poet. Soon after his birth, the Hovey family moved from Normal, where his father was president of the State Normal University, to the East Coast. He was raised primarily in Washington, DC, and graduated from Dartmouth College in 1885. Then he spent a year acting in amateur theatricals and studying in an Episcopal seminary. His first major work was *Launcelot and Guenevere* (1891), a series of plays based on the Arthurian cycle. In 1887 he met Canadian poet Bliss Carman, and they went on a walking tour of New England. His most noted book, *Songs from Vagabondia* (1894), was a collaboration with Carman. A popular

success, it was soon followed by *More Songs from Vagabondia*
(1896). During 1894 and 1895 Hovey lived abroad, first in England, where he translated the plays of Maurice Maeterlinck, and
then in France, where he was influenced by the Symbolists. In
1896 he returned to the United States, to live in Washington, DC,
and New York. Toward the end of the century, he wrote poems in
defense of the Spanish-American War and issued a collection of his
poetry, *Along the Trail* (1898). After teaching for a year at Barnard
College, he died in 1900 at age thirty-five.[35]

Hovey had a gift for creating rhythmically powerful lines, which
is apparent in "Unmanifest Destiny," a poem in support of the
Spanish-American War:

> To what new fates, my country, far
>   And unforeseen of foe or friend,
> Beneath what unexpected star,
>   Compelled to what unchosen end,
>
> Across the sea that knows no beach
>   The Admiral of Nations guides
> Thy blind obedient keels to reach
>   The harbor where thy future rides!
> . . . .
> There is a Hand that bends our deeds
>   To mightier issues than we planned;
> Each son that triumphs, each that bleeds,
>   My country, serves Its dark command.
>
> I do not know beneath what sky
>   Nor on what seas shall be thy fate;
> I only know it shall be high,
>   I only know it shall be great.[36]

"America" and "The Word of the Lord from Havana" are other
well-known poems that Hovey wrote in response to the war. He
was, then, a public poet, like so many others in the Illinois tradition.

One of Hovey's most interesting poems is a humorous piece
called "Her Valentine." It was written for the "new woman," whose

love had to be won in a way that did not compromise her individu-
ality:

> What, send her a valentine? Never!
> I see you don't know who "she" is.
> I should ruin my chances forever;
> My hopes would collapse with a fizz.[37]

The speaker goes on to characterize the new woman and to declare
that he doesn't want to restrict or dominate her: "I've no dream of
becoming her master,/ I've no notion of being her lord." But his
poem is, after all, an expression of male confidence that his wooing
will succeed:

> She may lecture (all lectures but curtain),
> Make money, and naturally spend;
> If I let her have her way, I'm certain
> She'll let me have mine in the end.

Unfortunately, Hovey's poetic vision was not complex or probing, and his technique was conventional. Nevertheless, his poems
often express his unconventional values, and that makes them
interesting reading for the student of late nineteenth-century
American literature.

William Vaughan Moody (1869-1910) was, in effect, the last
nineteenth-century Illinois poet, even though most of his poems
were published in the early years of the twentieth century, for his
poetic sensibility was deeply romantic and Victorian. Readers of
his poetry will note similarities to Keats, Browning, Morris, and
others. In his own time, Moody was regarded as a great American
poet and playwright, but as with Field and Hovey, his literary
reputation has declined.

Born and raised in Indiana, Moody graduated from Harvard in
1893 and received his M.A. degree there a year later. By the time
he joined the English faculty at the University of Chicago in 1895,
he had already been writing poetry for several years. Like Hovey,
he wrote verse dramas as well as lyrics in the closing years of the
century. His *Masque of Judgment* was published in 1900 and his

Poems appeared a year later. He also edited works by Milton, Pope, and other writers, but his most noted scholarly achievement was *A History of English Literature* (1902). Moody traveled extensively in Europe and lived for periods of time in the East and in southern California, but he continued to reside off and on in Chicago until the year of his death.

Moody's plays, especially *The Faith Healer* (1909) and *The Great Divide* (1911), are still regarded as having some importance in the history of American drama, but his best poems are more frequently read. Some of them were written in response to the Spanish-American War, but unlike Hovey's, they are poems of protest. At first, Moody viewed the conflict as a necessary fight for Cuban independence, but when American troops struggled to subjugate the Phillipines, he opposed American policy there. One of his most famous poems, "An Ode in Time of Hesitation," criticizes the debased morality of an America that has "stooped to cheat/ And scramble in the market-place of war."[39] A shorter and more effective anti-imperialist poem, "On a Soldier Fallen in the Phillipines," is a kind of mock funeral oration in which the fallen hero is unaware of his country's immoral policies:

> Let him never dream that his bullet's scream
> went wide of its island mark,
> Home to the heart of his darling land where she
> stumbled and sinned in the dark.[40]

Like Hovey, Moody was also a love poet. Several of his poems were inspired by Harriet Brainerd, an older woman whom he loved, idealized, and finally married. Perhaps the best is "A Prairie Ride." It expresses a sense of deep communion with the midwestern countryside, which the poet achieved during a horseback ride with her:

> I never knew how good
> Were those fields and happy farms,
> Till, leaning from her horse, she stretched her arms
> To greet and to receive them; nor for all
> My knowing, did I know her womanhood
> Until I saw the gesture understood.[41]

As Martin Halpern has pointed out, in this poem Harriet Brainerd becomes "a symbol of the essential procreative energy in nature and of the eternal female principle."[42] As a result of her companionship, Moody's remembered experience of "the prairie land/ Where I was born" becomes a kind of Wordsworthian recollection in tranquility – a lasting spiritual resource, not to mention a poetic inspiration.

"The Menagerie" is a very different work, a humorous dramatic monologue in which the mildly intoxicated speaker reflects on his evolutionary relationship to animals after viewing a circus menagerie. The poet accepts the post-Darwinian view of man's animal heritage, but at the same time, he deflates humanity's pride as the apparent darling of evolutionary progress:

> Helpless I stood among those awful cages;
> The beasts were walking loose, and I was bagged!
> I, I, the last product of the toiling ages,
> Goal of heroic feet that never lagged, –
> A little man in trousers, slightly jagged.[43]

This is Moody's finest poem, and it is one of the best poems ever written on the impact of evolution. If he had employed colloquial language more frequently, and had explored the inner life of modern man with more consistency, he might have produced a greater poetic achievement. As it is, he was the finest Illinois poet before the Chicago Renaissance.

The Illinois poets who preceded Lindsay, Masters, and Sandburg created an interesting and readable body of poetry, but too often they were imitative and simplistic. That is especially apparent if one reads their less successful poems, which were not discussed here. Even Moody was seldom original – although "The Menagerie" showed that he could be. He had perhaps as much talent as the Chicago Renaissance poets, but he was not as innovative. He wanted to be part of the great tradition of English-speaking poets, which he knew so well, but in a sense, he was stifled by that tradition. He did not find the language that would have made his voice unique and his poetry powerful, although he did write some effective poems. Hovey, despite his study of the French symbolists, apparently did not grasp the symbolizing function of poetry. He did not portray his consciousness; he asserted his views. He wrote poetry of statement, notable for its rhythmic vitality but devoid of subtlety or complexity. The same can be said for Field, who was primarily a writer of humorous and sentimental verse. "The Bibliomaniac's Prayer" was as close as he ever got to portraying his inner life. It is apparent that he viewed his poetry as entertainment rather than serious literary art.

Although Field, Hovey, and Moody did not take much poetic interest in Illinois culture, the earlier poets, who lived on the frontier, frequently did. Two of them – H. and Eliza Snow – produced substantial records of their experience in the West. Unfortunately, the latter was not a very penetrating poet, although she did reflect the emotional life of the Mormons during a difficult – and historically significant – period of time. H. had greater talent. He used poetry to analyze his experience and satirize frontier culture. He was also the most versatile Illinois poet before the Chicago Renaissance, employing a variety of poetic forms and techniques. But despite his self-appointed role as "The Sangamo Bard," his acquaintance with Illinois culture was limited. After all, he was a British expatriate and cosmopolitan traveler who simply resided in Springfield for a few years, took an interest in some aspects of local culture, and then moved on.

The frontier poets in Illinois had an opportunity to escape from conventional (eastern and British) literary practices by developing a straightforward style that was appropriate to the new reality of the West. But they failed to do that. John Howard Bryant, for example, wrote many romantic landscape poems in Illinois, but his language is so conventional that they could have been written in his native state of Massachusetts. They do not express the unique environment of the frontier.

Only John Hay, who grew up on the frontier and started writing his mature work after the Civil War, reflected the unique consciousness and language of western residents. His Pike County Ballads are still entertaining, and they read aloud very well. But his insight was limited because he had, by 1870, rejected the culture of his youth. Unlike Mark Twain, he succeeded in becoming a recognized part of the eastern cultural establishment – and he didn't long for the lost world of his boyhood along the Mississippi River. Hay tended to portray westerners as courageous but violent, outspoken but shallow – fit subjects for humorous poetry.

Lindsay, Masters, and Sandburg took their native culture more seriously. They identified with the Midwest; they saw themselves as Illinoisans. They were fascinated with Lincoln, inspired by John Peter Altgeld, impressed with the prairie landscape, and interested in the communities they came from and lived in. The Chicago Renaissance was not just a new departure in poetic technique or a revolution in the language of poetry. It was also an assertion that midwestern culture was significant.

But we should not regard Lindsay, Masters, and Sandburg as the earliest Illinois poets who are worth reading. That would be giving the Chicago Renaissance too much importance. The finest Illinois poets who came before them were among the most sensitive and perceptive people of their time in the Midwest, and they created some interesting and rewarding poems. As modern readers, our challenge is to share their insights and recognize their achievements.

Notes

1 John Knoepfle, "Poetry," in *A Reader's Guide to Illinois Literature*, ed. Robert C. Bray (Springfield: Illinois Secretary of State, 1985), p. 65.

2 The best biography of Bryant is Charles H. Brown's *William Cullen Bryant* (New York: Charles Scribner's Sons, 1971). The Bryant volume in the Twayne series is a helpful study of his achievement: Albert F. McLean, Jr., *William Cullen Bryant* (New York: Twayne, 1964). A good article about his involvement with Illinois is David J. Baxten's "William Cullen Bryant: Illinois Landowner," *Western Illinois Regional Studies*, 1 (1978), 1-14.

3 *The Knickerbocker Magazine* version of "The Prairies" was recently reprinted in *Illinois Literature: The Nineteenth Century*, ed. John E. Hallwas (Macomb: Illinois Heritage Press, 1986), pp. 68-69, and the quoted passage is from that anthology.

For discussions of the mythic aspect of the poem, see "The Garden Myth in 'The Prairies,' *Western Illinois Regional Studies*, 1 (1978), 15-26, and Paul A. Newlin, "*The Prairie* and 'The Prairies': Cooper's and Bryant's Views of Manifest Destiny," in *Wllliam Cullen Bryant and His America: Centennial Conference Proceedings 1878-1978*, ed. Stanley Brodwin, et al. (New York: AMS Press, 1983), pp. 27-38.

4 *Poetical Works of William Cullen Bryant* (New York: D. Appleton, 1909), p. 165.

5 The discovery of H. and the significance of his achievement are discussed in the Introduction to *The Poems of H.: The Lost Poet of Lincoln's Springfield* ed. John E. Hallwas (Peoria, IL: Ellis Press, 1982); pp. 1-41. That his name may have been John Hancock was indicated in the headnote to his poems in *Illinois Literature: The Nineteenth Century*, op. cit., p. 65.

6 *The Poems of H.*, p. 93.

7 *The Poems of H.*, p. 133.

8 *The Poems of H.*, p. 121.

9 *The Poems of H.*, p. 151.

10 The best source of information on Goudy is the "Introduction" to *The Poetical Remains of Dr. Robert Goudy* (Springfield: privately printed, 1842), pp. vii-xi, which was written by his brother Calvin.

11 *The Poetical Remains of Dr. Robert Goudy*, p. 48.

12 The poem has been recently reprinted in *Illinois Literature: The Nineteenth Century*, op. cit., pp. 119-120.

13 Gregg has been the subject of a biography: John E. Hallwas, *Thomas Gregg: Early Illinois Poet and Author*, Western Illinois Monograph Series, No. 2 (Macomb: Western Illinois University, 1983).

14 The poem has been recently reprinted in *Illinois Literature: The Nineteenth Century*, op. cit., p. 120.

15 As quoted in *Thomas Gregg*. op. cit., pp. 72-73.

16 For information about Snow, see *The Life and Labors of Eliza H. Snow Smith, with a Full Account of Her Funeral Services* (Salt Lake City: The Juvenile Instructor Office, 1888) and Maureen Ursenbach Beecher, "The Eliza Enigma: The Life and Legend of Eliza R. Snow," in *Essays on the American West, 1974-1975*, ed. Thomas G. Alexander; Charles Redd Monographs in Western History, No. 6 (Provo, Utah: Brigham Young Univ. Press, 1976), pp. 29-46. For a discussion of her poems, see John E. Hallwas, "The Midwestern Poetry of Eliza Snow," *Western Illinois Regional Studies*, 5 (1982), 136-45.

17 *Poems, Religious, Historical, and Political*, I (Liverpool: F. D. Richards, 1856), p. 7.

18 Ibid., p. 12.

19 Ibid., p. 143.

[20] The most thorough account of Bryant's life is E. R. Brown's "John Howard Bryant: A Biographical Sketch," which appears in *Life and Poems of John Howard Bryant* (Elmwood, IL: privately printed, 1894), pp. 5-42. For a discussion of his poetic achievement, see John E. Hallwas, "The Poetry of John Howard Bryant," *MidAmerica*, 7 (1980), 27-39.

[21] *Life and Poems of John Howard Bryant*, p. 126.

[22] Ibid., p. 189.

[23] Ibid., p. 153.

[24] Ibid., p. 160.

[25] Ibid., pp. 190-91.

[26] Hay was the subject of a Pulitzer Prize-winning biography: Tyler Dennett, *John Hay: From Poetry to Politics* (New York: Dodd, Mead, 1934). For a more recent discussion of his political career, see Howard I. Kushner, *John Milton Hay: The Union of Poetry and Politics* (Boston: Twayne, 1977).

[27] Two book-length studies of Hay's literary achievement have appeared: Robert L. Gale, *John Hay* (Boston: Twayne, 1978) and Kelly Thurman, *John Hay as a Man of Letters* (Reseda, CA: Mojave Books, 1974). See also John E. Hallwas, "The Varieties of Humor in John Hay's Pike County Ballads," *MidAmerica V* (1978), 7-18.

[28] *The Complete Poetical Works of John Hay* (Boston: Houghton Mifflin, 1916), p. 3.

[29] Ibid., pp. 6-9.

[30] Ibid., pp. 10-11.

[31] For biographical information about Field, see Robert Conrow, *Field Days: The Life, Times, and Reputation of Eugene Field* (New York; Charles Scribner's Sons, 1974), Charles H. Dennis, *Eugene Field's Creative Years* (Garden City, NY: Doubleday, Page, 1924), and Slason Thompson, *Eugene Field: A Study in Heredity and Contradictions*, 2 vols. (1901; rpt. New York: Beekman Publishers, 1974).

[32] *The Poems of Eugene Field* (New York: Charles Scribner's Sons, 1922), p. 455.

[33] Ibid., pp. 22-23.

[34] Ibid., p. 248.

[35] The most important studies of Hovey are William R. Linneman, *Richard Hovey* (Boston: Twayne, 1976) and Allan Houston Macdonald, *Richard Hovey: Man and Craftsman* (1957; rpt. New York: Greenwood Press, 1968).

[36] *Along the Trail* (1903; rpt. New York: AMS Press, 1969), pp. 16-17.

[37] *Last Songs from Vagabondia*, with Bliss Carman (Boston: Small, Maynard, 1900), p. 68.

[38] For an account of Moody's life, see Maurice F. Brown, *Estranging Dawn: The Life and Works of William Vaughan Moody* (Carbondale: Southern Illinois Univ.

Press, 1973). That book and the following work are the finest studies of Moody's poetry: Martin Halpern, *William Vaughan Moody* (New york: Twayne, 1964).

[39] *The Poems and Plays of William Vaughan Moody* (Boston: Houghton Mifflin, 1912), I, 19.

[40] Ibid., I, 30.

[41] Ibid., I, 147-48.

[42] Halpern, p. 141.

[43] *The Poems and Plays of William Vaughan Moody*, I, 64-65.

Tradition and Innovation in Twentieth-Century Illinois Poetry

Daniel L. Guillory
Millikin University

ANY ART FORM is the result of two inevitable forces always operating – consciously or unconsciously – on the receptive mind of the artist: tradition and innovation. These powerful forces determine the ultimate value and meaning of a work. Too much tradition can render a work bloodless and repetitive. Too much innovation can result in something that is so far ahead of its time that it misses its present audience altogether because it has no footing in the past and no hold on the future. Thus, the successful work of art is necessarily a delicate and precarious balancing of past and future, of tradition and innovation.

This artistic balancing or reconciliation of opposites is especially critical in the writing of poetry because language is the most utilized of civilized instruments and hence the most blunted. Yet the deepest and most evocative poems rely on the oldest and most traditional strengths of language – its tendency to create myth (*muthos*) and its uncanny ability to replicate the pictorial features of a locale (*ut pictura poesis*) and every nuance of the voices spoken there.[1]

Twentieth-century Illinois poetry began with Edgar Lee Masters' *Spoon River Anthology*, a work that balanced the traditional elements of monologue (a tradition going from Browning to the Classical Greeks) with a highly innovative verse form and ironic attitude. Of course, Edgar Lee Masters exerted a strong influence on all future poets. So Illinois poets of the twentieth century have been forced in a special way to heed these dialectical forces of tradition and innovation.

In practical terms, the use of tradition has meant an adherence to two kinds of icons: icons of place and icons of voice. Tradition means those elements of a culture which persist, and in Illinois the land and the voices spoken on it have been powerfully persistent and influential. In no other part of the world is space partitioned and organized in such a geometrical way as it is in Illinois, with its broad, 360-degree horizons, and silhouetted icons of barn, silo, and windmill. The spatial vastness sharpens the eye and forces close inspection of every vertical presence in this planar world.[2] In like manner, the great emptiness of place necessitated a great social emptiness, too. Early settlers were often cut off from one another, and Illinois speech developed a certain fidelity of description and brevity of expression because interlocutors experienced the world in those terms. Even today a poet living in the urban sprawl of Chicago can gain access to the prairie by a short drive on the interstate highway. Once there, the poet encounters a world of surreal emptiness, where, in the words of John Nims,

> No peak or jungle obscures the blue sky;
> Our land rides smoothly in the softest eye.[3]

Icons of place figure prominently in *Prairiescapes*, a splendid book of photographs by Illinois photographer Larry Kanfer.[4] In *Prairiescapes* Kanfer provides a virtual encyclopedia of the traditional icons of place in Illinois: the slatted corn cribs, the emerald green corn fields, the regal red barns, the silver-capped silos, and the spindly towers of windmills. These obsessive images of place inform all the arts, especially poetry. Illinois seems to breed poets with an unusually keen sense of place, as in this example from John Knoepfle's lyric "Saturday Morning," taken from his collection *Poems from the Sangamon*:

> the river is ditched here
> an interrupted line on the map
> still green to the eye though
> and crowding its slender grasses
> the old channel
> insinuates itself through cornfields
> loops across and back
> or coils alongside the ditch
> still roaming its old valley

telephone cables overhead
catch the gusts of a storm
the gray light of morning whines
you turn searching for something
that should be there.[5]

The land that is sung back into being in this poetry is not merely
the land of hedgerows and fence posts, John Deere tractors and
silver-black furrows. It is also the land of the Rust Belt, the land of
mid-sized industrial "feeder" towns, which supply parts for the
larger industrial complexes of St. Louis, Chicago, and Cleveland,
towns like Decatur, Illinois, as celebrated in John Knoepfle's
"Decatur":

they make everything in this
steam crowned city all these
air bearing crankshaft casings
easy ice cream scoops cardboard containers
made by hands laced with razor cuts
pasteurized ice milk and pumps and
imitation bacon bits who can say
from imitation hogs and corn sweeteners
and gear case housings stove knob inlays
creeper wheel assemblies potato chips
so many things here this very thingness
smolders in the whorls of our fingers.[6]

Knoepfle's technique of turning a catalogue of items into poetry
goes back as far as Homer and the ancient Greeks, but a more
recent source for this kind of traditional preoccupation in the
twentieth-century poetry of Illinois lies obviously in the work of
Carl Sandburg and especially in his long poem, *The People, Yes*,
with its litany of *homo faber*'s accomplishments:

Man the flint grinder, iron and bronze welder,
smoothing mud into hut walls,
smoothing reinforced concrete into
bridges, breakwaters, office buildings –
. . . .
waves, signals, buttons, sparks –
man with hands for loving and strangling,

man with the open palm of living handshakes,
man with the closed nails of the fist of combat –
these hands of man – where to? What next?[7]

And, of course, there could be no poem on Decatur, or
Bloomington, or Clinton, or New Berlin (some of the towns and
cities featured in Knoepfle's *Poems from the Sangamon*) without
that ur-poem of the modern city, Carl Sandburg's "Chicago," a
poem that boasts the improvisational complexity of a jazz composition, with the additive and repetitive feeling of successive floors
being built one atop the other, like those of a typical skyscraper
rising in the Loop. In its very structure, Sandburg's "Chicago" is
expressing the notion of the Infinite City: like a good jazz number
or a vaulting skyscraper, the poem can theoretically go on and on,
limited only by the energy and daring of its creator. Sandburg
virtually deifies the city by turning it into a kind of worker-god, a
sort of pugilistic *deus loci*, "laughing as a young man laughs,/
Laughing even as an ignorant fighter laughs who has never lost a
battle."[8] Such transcriptions of urban experience on a large scale
opened the way for more personal claims on the city, as in Lucien
Stryk's "A Sheaf for Chicago." In this moving, richly nostalgic
account of his childhood in the Windy City, Stryk splices together
nine separate but closely related poems about Chicago, including
"A Child in the City," which suggests the powerful poetic possibilities inherent in vacant lots and junkyards:

In a vacant lot behind a body shop

I rooted for your heart, O city,
The truth that was a hambone in your slop.

Your revelations came as thick as bees
With stings as smarting, wings as loud,
And I recall those towering summer days

We gathered fenders, axles, blasted hoods
To build Cockaigne and Never-never Land,
Then beat for dragons in the oily weeds.[9]

A more recent transcription of Chicago life, reflecting the gritty
urgencies of the contemporary scene, occurs in Michael Ananaia's
"News Notes, 1970":

and the bottles rocks flew
Grant Park the yachts still
lolling their slow dance of
masts and flying bridges
tear gas a few gunshots
evening papers tally the costs
in police cars fashionable windows
several injured none dead
fear a new alliance beginning
"the brothers and the longhairs"
"mellow," one said surprised.[10]

These icons of place, whether pastoral or urban, represent one –
but by no means the only – expression of tradition in Illinois
poetry of this century. Perhaps the most persistent expression of
tradition has come about through the various attempts to replicate
the icons of voice found in the region. By *voice* I don't mean simply
the dialectal particularity of a certain speaker, although dialectal
color is part of the voice. By voice I mean a set of attitudes and
postures; the voice is the way one claims the world, a subtle
appropriation of reality through unique stops and starts, syntacti-
cal leaps, and idiosyncratic phrasing. The voice is the grammar of
particularized experience. Edgar Lee Masters elevated the poetry
of voice (and simultaneously put Illinois on the poetry map of
America) by publishing *Spoon River Anthology* in 1915.[11] Although
Masters plundered *The Greek Anthology* for the fundamentally
ironic tone and retrospective stance of his speakers, their voices
are the pure products of the prairie. In one of the most famous
monologues, "Margaret Fuller Slack," one hears the plaintive and
embittered voice of a woman who would have lived an infinitely
richer life, she believes, if only fate had been kinder. The poem
contains at least four distinct breaks in thought and mood – sig-
nalled on the page by uneven line lengths, a dash, a question mark,
and a strategically placed, terminal exclamation point:

I would have been as great as George Eliot
But for an untoward fate.
For look at the photograph of me made by Penniwit,

Chin resting on hand, and deep-set eyes –
Gray, too, and far-searching.
But there was the old, old problem:
Should it be celibacy, matrimony or unchastity?
Then John Slack, the rich druggist, wooed me,
Luring me with the promise of leisure for my novel,
And I married him, giving birth to eight children,
And had no time to write.
It was all over with me, anyway,
When I ran the needle in my hand
While washing the baby's things,
And died from lock-jaw, an ironical death.
Hear me, ambitious souls,
Sex is the curse of life![12]

The agony, the self-pity, the remorse, the imagination of Margaret Fuller (those names a suggestion of her assertiveness and talent) Slack (that surname an emblem of her drab environment) all come to life in that voice. In fact, *Spoon River Anthology* is a supreme collection of voices, not real street voices but artificially enhanced, hybridized versions of the village argot. Art always transforms and intensifies its subjects. Masters uses death as a shortcut for this artistic enhancement of speech; Margaret Fuller Slack may speak freely because, like all the other voices from Spoon River, she is dead. The poetic use of voice continues to assert itself most powerfully in the most recent poetry of the region. In John Knoepfle's *Poems from the Sangamon*, for example, one hears this marvelous specimen of rural Illinois yawp, full of wry humor and the characteristic intonations of the Heartland. The poem is entitled "Watching a Haircut," and the poet functions here as editor and transcriber of these little gems of rural speech:

they don't put you down
six feet anymore
just forty-two inches
say thats enough now
why its hardly below frost
well they say you can't heave out
the vaults a ton and a half

and what about the water table
how about we get rain for a month
I ask them that and they say
well one did rise up
on polecat creek near Chatham
last year first of March
but they was an admiral in it
so it was all right.[13]

In a similar vein, one hears a disturbing and effective pathos and
irony in "Pauline Bites Her Thread in Two, Then Says" from
Katherine Kerr's *First Frost*:

First I ever learned about sex
was from an old medical text:
Problems in Obstetrics.
Every misformed pelvis possible
was pictured there.
Hemmorhoids, hernia, hydrocephalus –
you got it – tumors, twin pipes . . .
I married late. Worked a month waitressing
right after the wedding. Chili-mac
was the cheapest thing on the menu –
you know, beans and runny sauce
over spaghetti noodles.
Only serving I ever saw
came back. Came back up, that is,
on the old wino who laid his face
down in it before he left.
For a dollar an hour and tips
I cleaned it up,
fearing I'd have syphillis
from touching his "bodily fluids."
And since he'd left without paying
the cashier took the tip.[14]

The fact that Pauline has been "short-changed" on her whole life
is fully suggested in this wry anecdote. Pauline belongs to the same
world as Duane Taylor's Parley Porter, who, in *Family Scraps: Ten
Poems in the Voice of Parley Porter*, reveals the touching inti-

macies of his life, including his complex feelings for his mother ("Parley's Mother is Extolled") who tamed an ox one winter:

> She beat a lively
> load of rugs at eighty-five
> and died one Thursday squeezing
> the teats of her best cow
> Her stone says *Like merchant ships*
> *she bringeth food from afar.* [15]

The one poet who has inherited Edgar Lee Masters' knack for using voice in all its possibilities is Dave Etter, as suggested in his little book, *Cornfields*, and particularly in a poem like "Rudy Gerstenberg: Memo to the Erie-Lackawanna":

> If there was ever a boxcar
> with its pants down, so to speak,
> your old 68401 was it, all right.
> Both doors were slung open wide
> and some clown had written the usual
> "clean me" and "Kilroy was here."
> Now, I want you to know, too,
> I'm in love with Erie-Lackawanna.
> But beat-up 68401 sure let me down,
> and I ended up feeling railroaded all day. [16]

All of these voices (notably those created by Knoepfle, Kerr, Taylor, and Etter) are voices just one stroke short of despair. In a world where most characters – and the authors who create them – are required to maintain a stiff upper lip, these poetic voices are refreshingly honest and expressive about the pain that always circumscribes human experience. Perhaps these barbers, farmers, and waitresses possess a simplicity that is also a kind of freedom; perhaps they do not *know* how to dissemble, especially to themselves. Hence, they become especially valuable to their poet-creators since they serve as mouthpieces to speak of things most vulnerable and tender in everyday human life.

Icons of voice and icons of places are, thus, the most obvious expressions of tradition in Illinois poetry. Tradition depends upon a whole welter of unconscious assumptions about what is important, where to begin, and where to stop. Without tradition, there could be no art. Yet without its polar opposite of innovation, tradition would become ossified and sterile. If tradition can be thought of as the common mind of a culture, then innovation is the expression of individual needs within that more general framework.

The poets writing in Illinois after the Great Depression and the Second World War brought to their artistry a particular kind of refinement that in many ways superseded the stunning but rather facile break-throughs of the pioneering trio (Masters, Sandburg, and Lindsay). One way of describing the difference between the poets writing actively after mid-century and those who wrote before that benchmark is to call the more recent poets aestheticist – that is, poets whose primary concern is the enhancement of feeling (one receives an *anæsthetic* to prevent feeling during surgery or tooth extractions).

An aestheticist preoccupation reveals itself in the finest work of Gwendolyn Brooks, Lisel Mueller, Lucien Stryk, Michael Ananaia, and Laurence Lieberman, even though all of these poets have, on occasion, written the more traditional sort of Illinois poem. The important difference in the newer poetry is the kind of mind brought to bear upon the work. A delicacy and subtlety of perception typifies the new poems, as if the poets were working with fine, laser-like instruments while their predecessors hacked away with crude hand tools of metal and stone.

This tendency toward aesthetic enhancement is not to be confused with a desire for "prettiness" or postcard cuteness in a work. It can best be described as a supreme effort of focusing, a minute examination of a particular, as in Gwendolyn Brooks' "The Sundays of Satin-Legs Smith." Here, she focuses on his outlandish zoot suit, a kind of metaphor for the extravagant psychological suitings all citizens wear, even those who are not pimps or residents of Bronzeville, like Mr. Smith:

> Let us proceed. Let us inspect, together
> With his meticulous and serious love,
> The innards of this closet. Which is a vault

Whose glory is not diamonds, not pearls,
Not silver plate with just enough dull shine.
But wonder-suits in yellow and in wine,
Sarcastic green and zebra-striped cobalt.
With shoulder padding that is wide
And cocky and determined as his pride;
Ballooning pants that taper off to ends
Scheduled to choke precisely.
                                        Here are hats
Like bright umbrellas; and hysterical ties
Like narrow banners for some gathering war. [17]

Here Miss Brooks makes art by discovering her subject – a South
Side pimp – *as* a work of art. And the resultant poem moves into a
new field that transcends its initial social commentary and
documentary coverage. The poem begins to play with language
and luxuriate in it; colors become dazzling unto themselves. An
aestheticist, not merely a regional or even ethnic, poem has been
born. Likewise, in Lisel Mueller's "The Power of Music to Disturb," a magnificent poem about love, death, and the mediation of
music between these two extremes, one delights in domestic details
while being instructed (as only a poem can instruct) about the
aesthetic potency of music:

My God, he was a devil of a man
who wrote this music so voluptuous
it sucks me in with possibilities
of sense and soul, of pity and desire
which place and time make ludicrous: I sit
across from you here in our living room
with chairs and books and red geraniums
and ordinary lamplight on the floor
after an ordinary day of love. [18]

In its language and its sophisticated juxtapositions of the com-
monplace and the sublime, Mueller's poem makes the reader appreciate the irony of that final phrase "ordinary day of love." Every
day of love is extraordinary, every day itself is extraordinary, and
music exists to suggest these profound and gratifying discoveries.

This introduction of another art form – music – really, another frame of reference, is altogether typical of the more innovative poetry to come out of Illinois, especially in the last two decades. A poet might very well derive inspiration from a totally different environment, philosophy, or point of view, as in the example of Lucien Stryk, whose work has been dramatically changed by his contact with Zen artists and poets during his many visits to Japan, where he worked on various translations of Japanese Zen poetry. In "Making Poetry," an essay he wrote for William Heyen's important anthology, *American Poets in* 1976, Stryk describes the profound effect of Zen on the composition of one of his major (although relatively early) poems, "Zen: The Rocks of Sesshu." The poet recalls how he told a famous Zen master "some very stupid things about the rock garden." The Zen master responded that he must look at the garden "with the navel," an injunction that left the poet with an "acute self-disgust." Determined to write a new kind of poem, Stryk abandons his earlier drafts of the poem about the rock garden:

> Working for hours without a break, I transformed the poem I had been writing on the garden, ridding it of "filling," breaking down rigidly regular stanzas, a welter of words, to a few "image units" of around two and one-half lines, while keeping to a constant measure, the short line throughout being of the same syllabic length. In fact, though unintended, the stanzaic unit I came up with was in length and feeling very close to the haiku, and at its best as compact as the short Zen poems I was translating.[19]

The meditational act of Zen and the rational program of translating Zen poetry became an intimate part of Stryk's compositional technique, the result of which is beautifully evident in this fourth (of eight) sections in the poem:

> Who calls her butterfly
> Would elsewhere
> Pardon the snake its fangs:
>
> In the stony garden
> Where she flits
> Are sides so sharp, merely

To look gives pain. Only
    The tourist,
Kodak aimed and ready for

The blast, ship pointing for the
    Getaway,
Dare raise that parasol.[20]

In a more recent poem, "Awakening" (which is dedicated to Ha-
kuin, Zen master of the late seventeenth and early eighteenth
century), Stryk uses the Zen technique of "mind-pointing" to
focus, first on a sumi-e (ink-brush) painting, then to focus on
Illinois scenes, particularly changes in the light and weather. The
poem comes to an extraordinary summation in its final (seventh)
section when the poet is literally absorbed by his environment.
The Japanese meditational practice has been fully appropriated
and applied to the haunting openness of the prairie at sunset:

I write in the dark again,
rather by dusk-light,
and what I love about
this hour is the way the trees
are taken, one by one,
into the great wash of darkness.

At this hour I am always happy,
ready to be taken myself,
fully aware.[21]

Awareness of the kind Stryk achieves at the close of this poem is
facilitated by another frame of reference, here Zen meditation, but
other frames of reference have proven to be powerful inspirations
for contemporary poetry. John Knoepfle, for example, has been
mightily inspired by his study of the Illinois Indian languages
(such as the Tamaroa and Peoria), by his transcriptions of oral
history gathered along the Ohio River, and by his close study of the
early history of Illinois, which inspired poems on Marquette and
Peter Cartwright, among others. Still another – and surprising – frame of reference for Knoepfle is that of geological history,

which allows him to do an altogether new kind of poem about the
Illinois prairie, as shown in these stanzas from "Soundings in
Glacial Drift" (from *Poems from the Sangamon*):

> at the county line road
> the macon and christian county divide
> there is a benchmark
> copper green on a culvert wall
> it is precisioned
> at the intersected baseline
> of the third principal meridian
> this is the interior of our interior
> pending from the numeraled stars
>
> south of this place
> through walls of dust
> you can see glacial kames
> sucked from wisconsin meltdowns
> the ice two miles high then
> think of it.[22]

For Laurence Lieberman, a poet who has lived in Illinois for
many years without being preoccupied with Illinois as a subject
per se, the frame of reference becomes paramount in importance,
and for Lieberman that frame is either Japan or the Caribbean. In
his most major work, *Eros at the World Kite Pageant, Poems* 1979-
1982, Lieberman writes entire sequences of poems about these
places, as, for example, the complex work entitled "The Kashi-
kojima Quartet." From another section of the book called "Song of
Leave-Taking" comes "Loves of the Peacock," a poem very much
in the manner of Marianne Moore (whom Lieberman admires
extremely and whose syllabic verse form he uses exhaustively).
This poem is a quintessentially aestheticist treatment of the
peacock, a minute examination of the bird's particularities. It is a
minor triumph, a poem that in the best sense of the term is entirely
modernist:

> The male peafowl
> opens and closes his iridescent wings,
>   slowly, rising on his toes;
>   his chest swells, his wings a pump
>   or bellows inflating his trunk and lengthy abdomen,

> by gradual puffs. We hear
> a faint hissing . . .
> He squints his eyes, and swiftly unfolds
> the many loose webs
> of his gorgeously elongated tail plumes
> into a broad half-moon-shaped aquamarine fan![23]

Michael Ananaia uses a complex set of historical references clustered around the Lewis and Clark expedition to create a frame of reference for the long poem "The Riversongs of Arion" in *Riversongs*. In addition to this historical frame, Ananaia uses a complex, rather French attitude toward the work. There is a deconstructionist quality to some of the poems (like the ninth song of Arion) that at some point recalls the work of Barthes, Lacan, and Derrida:

> The sunlight on the water,
> landfall shadows, treeline
> edging down the slow current.
>
> This is the land I made for you
> by hand, what was touched once
> then misremembered into words,
>
> place where the soil slips out
> from under its trees, where
> stiff weeds fall like rapids.[24]

What makes this poem innovative – and appealingly so – is its rather self-conscious artistry, its tendency to call attention to itself and to the process of interpreting itself. The "land" has a basis in external reality but is clearly the product of the poet's imagination which "misremembers" everything "into words." The poem tells its audience that it is only a poem, yet in the boldness of that declaration lies an even greater poem, as if the poet can reveal much because he realizes an even larger (though undefined) something remains secret and untouched.

A recent poem by Bruce Guernsey, "The Phone Booth" from his chapbook *The Invention of the Telephone*, combines the self-conscious artistry and surprising frame of reference (here, the philosophical difficulty of communication, especially of uttering "I love you") with an ordinary prairie setting to produce a powerful and memorable poem:

> Today
> by a one pump station
> in some cornfield town
> I said I love you
> on the phone, words
> I haven't said
> to anyone for years
> or written down
> but had to stop
> in a dry wind
> in a flat place
> to say, to say
> I love you
> clear and sure
> out of the wind
> in the rattling glass
> of a phone booth,
> a place perhaps
> to start again
> where gray wings whirl
> above the bins
> hollow, hollow,
> and the tall grass bends.[25]

Idea and image merge beautifully here; the man needs the empty place to act out his own emptiness; he needs the distancing of the telephone to say what is nearest to his heart (in fact, "Long Distance," might have been an equally suitable, if more obvious, title). And, finally, the man who has been too, too, proud finally learns to "bend," just like the tall grass that so graphically defines the prairie.

As Bruce Guernsey's poem eloquently demonstrates, contemporary Illinois poets are still grappling – successfully, in this instance – with the forces of innovation and tradition. Guernsey's poem is entirely modern, with its spare, minimalist phrasing and its deep interiorizing of experience, but the poet fashions for himself an icon of voice that echoes some of the lonelier utterances from *Spoon River Anthology*. And the content (or message) of that voice is inseparable from the icons of place (phone booth, grain silo, prairie grass) that serve as literal and metaphorical meanings. Voice and place are tightly wedded; tradition and innovation, the shaping forces of Illinois poetry, are reconciled once again (as they have been over and over in the past 75 years) in that supreme balancing act we call poetry.

Notes

[1] See Ernst Cassirer, "The Place of Language and Myth in the Pattern of Human Culture" in *Language and Myth*, trans. Susanne K. Langer (New York: Dover, 1953), pp. 1-17.

[2] In *Songlines* (New York: Viking, 1987), Bruce Chatwin explains how the Aborigines have turned the entire continent of Australia into a kind of mythic map, with all key topographical features connected by "songlines" or long, poetic narratives. And on p. 52, Chatwin explains that "an unsung land is a dead land."

[3] John F. Nims, "Midwest," in *Heartland: Poets of the Midwest*, ed. Lucien Stryk (DeKalb: Northern Illinois University Press, 1967), p. 150.

[4] See Larry Kanfer, *Prairiescapes* (Urbana: University of Illinois Press, 1987).

[5] John Knoepfle, *Poems from the Sangamon* (Urbana: University of Illinois Press, 1985), p. 5.

[6] Knoepfle, *Poems from the Sangamon*, p. 30.

[7] Carl Sandburg, *Harvest Poems*, ed. Mark Van Doren (New York: Harcourt, Brace, Jovanovich, 1960) pp. 102-103.

[8] Carl Sandburg, *Harvest Poems*, p. 35.

[9] Lucien Stryk, *Collected Poems* (Chicago: Swallow, 1984), p. 23.

[10] Michael Ananaia, *Riversongs* (Urbana: University of Illinois Press, 1978), p. 45.

[11] Edgar Lee Masters, *Spoon River Anthology* (1915; rpt. New York: Collier, 1962, with intro. by May Swenson).

[12] Masters, *Spoon River Anthology*, p. 70.

[13] Knoepfle, *Poems from the Sangamon*, p. 38.

[14] Kathryn Kerr, *First Frost* (Urbana: Stormline Press, 1985), p. 81.

[15] Duane Taylor, *Family Scraps: Ten Poems in the Voice of Parley Porter* (Urbana: Stormline Press, 1986), p. 12.

[16] Dave Etter, *Cornfields*(Peoria: Spoon River Press, 1980), p. 18.

[17] Gwendolyn Brooks, "The Sundays of Satin-Legs Smith," in *Heartland*, p. 16.

[18] Lisel Mueller, "The Power of Music to Disturb," *Heartland*, p. 148.

[19] Lucien Stryk, "Making Poetry," in *American Poets in 1976*, ed. William Heyen (Indianapolis: Bobbs Merrill, 1976), p. 393.

[20] Stryk, *Collected Poems*, p. 45.

[21] Stryk, *Collected Poems*, p. 108.

[22] Knoepfle, *Poems from the Sangamon*, p. 52.

[23] Laurence Lieberman, *Eros at the World Kite Pageant, Poems 1979-1982* (New York: Macmillan, 1983), p. 26.

[24] Ananaia, *Riversongs*, p. 20.

[25] Bruce Guernsey, *The Invention of the Telephone* (Urbana: Stormline Press, 1987), p. 12.

OBAC and the Black Chicago Poets:
Towards a Black Visual Aesthetic*

Maria K. Mootry
Grinnell College

What is poetry? It is the human soul entire, squeezed like a lemon or lime, drop by drop, into automatic words . . . Hang yourself, poet, in your own words. Otherwise you are dead.[1]
– Langston Hughes

We want live words of the hip world live flesh & coursing blood. Hearts Brains Souls splintering fire. We want poems like fists.[2]
– Imamu Amiri Baraka

THROUGHOUT their mid-century poetic careers, the triumvirate of modernist Black poets, Gwendolyn Brooks, Robert Hayden, and Melvin Tolson, were known for their versatile poetic technique and their ability to shift from classical to vernacular diction and forms. In their massive shadow, the Black poets of the sixties, including the poets associated with the Chicago workshop OBAC (Organization of Black American Culture), seem to be found wanting. OBAC poets, and Black Aesthetic poets in general, have been accused of lacking any sense of craft because their overriding sociopolitical ideology seemed to preclude the modernist's concern for Art. Accused of being indiscriminate in their acceptance of all writing as long as it supported a black ideology, Chicago's OBAC poets, and all Black Aesthetic poets of the sixties, might be better understood as artists who sought to expand the modernist project of dismantling boundaries within and among the arts, just as they sought to dismantle what they perceived

*A shorter version of this paper appeared under the title, "The OBAC Tradition: Don L. Lee, Carolyn Rodgers and The Early Years," in Carole Parks' anthology, *NOMMO*. Tom Mitchell's 1988 NEH Summer Seminar on "The Verbal and the Visual" helped me during the revision and enlargement of the essay. Finally, enthusiastic comments from my colleague, Michael Bell, encouraged me to refine and clarify several assertions in the paper.

61

as unjust social and political boundaries. In the context of black and white, national and international, counterculture and street culture movements that dominated the sixties, certainly, black sixties poets felt freer than Black modernists to push language into an open field, aurally and visually. And certainly their use of "profane" words and street language in general makes the modernist shift from "high" to "low" diction seem tame in comparison. Carolyn Rodgers, an OBAC poet, would begin a poem with the lines "I mah/kick yo ass-ss/" without blinking; and one of the most productive popular OBAC poets, Don L. Lee (now Haki Madhubuti), could report his girlfriend's opinion of men – "blackmen ain't shit" – with similar lack of compunction.

In fact, much of the poetry of Chicago Black poets and OBAC poets employed visual as well as verbal "transgressions" of traditional poetic language. Visual shapes, visual puns and other visual "shocks" were added to oral, aural and semantic dimensions of their texts as these writers struggled, not only with the racially provincial issue of what constitutes a Black Aesthetic, but with the abiding and more formally modernist questions of the relationship between word and image, being and language, poetic theory and poetic practice.

In the 1960s, Black Chicago poets and other artists seemed to live in a charged environment, a convulsive present, a "nowtime" enlivened by the dialectic of their individual talents and cataclysmic local and national events that included Civil Rights activities, urban riots, assassinations, and the rise of a Black Power movement. While they addressed these issues, the poets' artistic practice was nourished and honed by numerous groups at numerous sites, including the South Side Community Art Center, the Du Sable Museum of Afro-American History, Phil Cohran's Afro-Arts Theatre, Ellis' Bookstores, Val Gray Ward's Kuumba Workshop (theatre), and the Organization of Black American Culture (OBAC). Founded in the spring of 1967 by mentor-editor Hoyt Fuller, black intellectual Gerald McWorter (Abdul Alkalimat) and poet Conrad Kent Rivers, OBAC was initially divided into an artist's workshop and a writer's workshop. While the artists broke off to form Afri-Cobra, the OBAC writers' workshop flourished on its own, publishing a journal, *NOMMO*, and meeting weekly to nurture local talent and share works with nationally known writers who were passing through the Windy City. After meeting at the Southside Community Art Center and the Du Sable Museum, the group settled into a "home" at 77 East 35th Street. Gwendolyn Brooks, Pulitzer Prize winner and state poet-laureate, soon became an avid mentor of the group, helping to give it visibility and to make it one of the most influential workshops in the country. In its twenty-year history, OBAC helped some of the most prolific young Black writers today, including Angela Jackson, Haki R. Madhubuti, David L. Crockett-Smith, Mike Cook, and Sterling Plumpp.[3]

Charged with the challenge to present the "infinite subtlety, variety, complexity, and substance" of the Black experience,[4] the OBAC poets not only wrote poems but penned essays, clarified issues, and took stands in the swirling debate over the form and function of art. In the process, they consciously confronted what David Antin has separated out as the "conservative wing" of American modernist poetry, i.e., the Metaphysical Modern Tradition with its origins in some of the work by Pound, Eliot, and Stevens.[5] According to Antin, modernism itself very early divided into two strains: the Pound-Eliot-Stevens variety and a "purer" modernism that was more "open" in form and social persuasion. This "purer" modernism was, in part, located in the visual aspect of Pound's poetic practice. It was the purer modernism, progressing from Pound's ideograms and Appolinaire's calligrammes to the works of William Carlos Williams, Louis Zukofsky, Charles Olson, the Black Mountain Poets, the Beats, and the New York School, which would embrace a LeRoi Jones, editor of *Yugen*, who in turn would go on to become the most famous of the 1960s Black Aesthetic poets under the name Imamu Amiri Baraka. This is not (although it may be) a question of influence, but of conviction. In practice and ideology, the Chicago Black poets seem heavily influenced by Baraka, whom they admired and with whom they frequently performed. Even more than Baraka, they were convinced that writing poetry involved a "shifting view of the relation between text and poem." This aesthetic theory caused them to shift aesthetic emphasis in separate and sometimes complementary directions. One direction was toward an aural/oral asethetic that stressed performance and a speech/ear matrix with the multivocal sounds of street speech and popular culture. Another direction was towards a visual "eye" matrix, reified in the extreme by what had become known among modernists as Concrete poetry, where the poem was primarily image and/or design.

If, on a conceptual level, writing communicated the Black Chicago poets' consciousness; on a phenomenological level, paper and ink was their site of conflict and becoming. Richard Wright, another Chicago writer, had long ago described the black man as America's metaphor, but for the Black poets, writing itself was a metaphor of global racial struggle, reified in the very fact and act of the artist placing "black ink on white paper."[6] This was no retreat into either ambiguity or ideology, but an almost Bergsonian sense of becoming, a Fanonian sense of possibility, a Nietzschean sense of the transvaluation of values so that what was formerly "order" is seen as transgression and what is labeled transgression becomes a new order. For Don L. Lee (now known as Haki Madhubuti), for example, all poetic practice was fluid since a specific definition could "exclude improvement, advancement and change."[7]

For other OBAC poets like Carolyn Rodgers, artistic theory seemed less protean. Clear-cut "correct" and "incorrect" choices had to be made. In 1970, Rodgers denounced "White English" in her essay, "The Literature of Black," when she wrote:

> Black writers must not use the colonizer language as it exists. Correctness, learnedness, is intensified oppression, better oppression.[8]

Possibly following Frantz Fanon's remarks on the role of language in Afro-World oppression, Rodgers denounces not only "correct" pronunciation of English, but "correct" spelling, punctuation, and typography. Calling for a new order, she warns:

> To start sentences with capitals, to end sentences with periods, to use commas, etc., etc., etc., reeks of a higher subtler more destruc-

tive order. Which we seek to destroy in Black minds for example. (Rodgers, p. 10)

Even in her prose, Rodgers tries to defy what she considers language-oppressions. Writing "Black" for Carolyn Rodgers and for many other OBAC members, meant creating a new linguistic order: "call it flat rappin or round or rhyme rappin, dig it . . ." (Rodgers, p. 11). Rising to an almost mystical conclusion in her essay, Rodgers cites Coltrane's and Sun-Ra's non-European sound patterns as the basis for limitless forms, whether in poetry or the plastic arts. Painters, she suggests, should "forget canvases and paint on anything, everything." (Rodgers, p. 11). Perhaps it is no coincidence that Rodgers' first volume is titled *Paper Soul* (1968) because she seems to have a hyper-awareness of the materiality of writing, as this passage from the same essay indicates:

> the very order of words on paper becomes questionable . . . symptoms of the honkie's ORDER, like where you put stamps on letters how a man and woman walk down the street what fingers you wear rings on when married what time the world goes to work (9) and lunch 12-1 and gets off (5) . . . Perhaps what is needed is nonsense to create newsense. Liberating sense. Sense that has no oppressing tradition. Check. The very sentence, *John walked*, is totally different from John split, John made it, John spaced. (Rodgers, p. 6)

Ironically, while Rodgers seemed to place greater emphasis on disruption and revolution through changing artistic practice, Lee, who soon became a political poet-prophet like Baraka on the East coast, placed less emphasis on the efficacy of social change through art. For Lee, social change was imbedded primarily in alternative institutions like his Institute for Positive Education and his Third World Press. Yet it was Lee who pushed experiments in the verbal and visual farther than any of the other OBAC poets, including Rodgers.

Experiments with verbal and visual co-expressibility by OBAC poets took many forms. Looking at poems published in selective

texts such as the anthology *Jump Bad*, in Lee's three chapbooks
and in the commemorative volume, *To Gwen with Love*, a number
of strategies stand out.[9] On a macro-level, the poem as visible
shape or icon occurs, ironically recalling seventeenth-century
poems for the eye like Herbert's "Easter Wings." More frequently
the poets alter conventions of typography, changing customary
upper case letters to lower case and vice versa. Other visual
mechanics include the manipulation of white space and the poetic
line, and the use of internal visual patterning. Supra-semantic
indicators such as italics, asterisks, ampersands, slashes, and
dashes are also common. Certain orthographical usages recur
which reflect journalistic usage, such as "nite" for "night," or
"thru" for "through." On the other hand, usages such as "wd" for
"would," "u" for "you," and "blk" for "black" are reminiscent of
e.e. cummings' modernist visual poetry. Some of this usage co-ex-
presses the aural text, following Baraka's example when he wrote
in his poem, "Black Art," that what was needed was "Airplane
poems:

    rrrrrrrrrrrrrrrrrrrrrrrrrrrrrrrrrrrrrrr . . .

    tuhtuhtuhtuhtuhtuhtuhtuhtuh . . .

    rrrrrrrrrrrrrrrrrrrrrrrrrrrrrrrrrrrrrrr . . ."

Most interesting to this study are texts in which the visual and
the verbal merge in almost equal coexpressibility. For example, in
her poem about the anxiety of growing up black and female on
Chicago's Southside ("Remember Times for Sandy"), Carolyn
Rodgers asks, "where could the heart hide that beat SO
LOUDDDDDDDD?" (*Jump Bad*, p. 118). Some critics of the
Black Arts Movement found such usage gratuitous, even repellent.
However, it may be argued that here traditional paralinguistic
features of aural speech are yoked with visual form so that the
eight upper case D's represent not only the idea of loudness but,
among other interpretations, the repetitive sound of the anxiously
beating heart. A similar, more complex strategy is found in Rodgers' tour de force of verbal/visual poetry, "Somebody Call (for
help)," (*Jump Bad*, pp. 119-121). In this poem, the victimization of
a woman curiously parallels Herbert's poem about Christ's

crucifixion mentioned earlier. Herbert's famous visual poem conveys Christ's diminution, death, and rebirth in these expanding and contracting lines:

> Lord, who createdst man in wealth and store,
>   Though foolishly he lost the same,
>   Decaying more and more
>   Till he became
>   Most poor:
>   With thee
>   O let me rise
>   As larks, harmoniously,
> And sing this day thy victories:
> Then shall the fall further the flight in me.[10]

Visually, this stanza forms the shape of the wings in flight, if looked at horizontally; while vertically it suggests an altar made of two pyramids, one inverted atop the other.

Rodgers' poem also begins with two inverted pyramids which invite interpretation. As in Herbert's poem there is the visualization of a victim's destruction when the poem begins:

> i remember the night
> he beat
> her
> we all heard her scream
> him break some glass
> her beg

Several lines later the text highlights the rise and fall of a fist with the capitals impacting on the eye as a hand might on flesh: "beat HIM he beat HER beat HIM down the stairs." While Herbert's poem turns on the optimistic Christian paradox that a downward motion ("fall") would lead to redeeming upward motion ("further flight"), in Rodgers' poem, downwardness is stressed visually without redirection, but with accretion and expansion. Thus, it is when the police are called to help that ironically violence escalates into the pattern "beat HIM he beat HER beat him." Here is domestic life out of control, eliciting more violence from the forces of law and order. Rodgers' poem crescendoes thematically and

visually into a stunning final thirteen lines that *look* hysterical in
their visual patterning, with capital letters suggesting wild emotions, and capital "S's" and small "s's" suggesting the flow of
blood down the wall. The small "s's" turn to capital "S's" as the
violence escalates and the flow widens to include all Blacks who
fight one another, as in the recently ended Nigerian Civil War. The
single word "BLOOD" becomes almost a tragic logo, since it is a
pun, referring not only to destruction of life but ironically also
referring to Black people who called one another "blood" in affec-
tionate street slang. Here, to use McLuhanesque terminology, the
medium truly becomes the message; the poem is its cruel image,
with the final lines embodying severance and disjunction, the
asterisks becoming spots of black blood on the white page:

> BLOODSsss
> RUNNING RUNNING RUNNING
> against the walls
> BLOODSssss
> RUNNING RUNNING RUNNING
> in hall ways
>   BLOODDDSSS
> RUNNING RUNNING   RUNNING
>   THROUGHOUT THE WORLD
>   CUT*TING IN*TO EACH OTHER
>   some   body   (pleeease)
>   CALL
>   for help)

As proof of the success of the verbal/visual aesthetic, perhaps it
is no coincidence that the most quoted, memorized and enjoyed
Chicago Black poet, Don L. Lee, stretched poetry beyond its
bonds from verbal virtuosity into both visual and aural wit and
creativity. The street aesthetics of signifying, the jazz aesthetics of
riffing, and the oral tradition of "wolfing" or playing "bad" are
imaged in Lee's visual bravado and insouciance. In the concluding
poem of *Think Black!* Lee, as purveyor of a new way of looking
(and therefore thinking) about things, issues this "concrete" message which can be read horizontally as well as vertically:

```
BLACK      PEOPLE     THINK
PEOPLE     BLACK      PEOPLE
THINK      PEOPLE     THINK
BLACK      PEOPLE     THINK
THINK      BLACK.
```
(*Think Black!*, p. 24)

The spacing of this poem invites varied aural and semantic interpretation. Choices for cæesura, full stops, and alternative units of meaning are increased in this virtual ideogram. As arbiter of conscience, shaman, and artifact maker, Lee has provided simultaneously a hypnotic chant similar to the "OM" of Eastern devotees and a sampler to be framed and hung like a Chinese print. On the other hand, in "Mwilu/or Poem for the Living (for Charles and LaTanya)," Lee uses what may be called a visual jazz aesthetic, riffing on the page, sculpting a form out of a free-form aura. The poem, another cautionary text, begins:

```
jump   bigness   upward
like u jump clean    make everyday the weekend
& work like u party.
```
(*Jump Bad*, p. 40)

As the poem progresses, the visual element becomes more patterned, programmatic, and integrated with the message, defying traditional usage to its own aural and visual ends:

```
never   Muslim eating pig sandwiches   never
never   listerine breath even cuss proper   never
never   u ignorant because smart was yr teacher   never
never   wander under wonder fan-like avenues.   never
never   will be never as long as never teaches   never.
```
(*Jump Bad*, p. 41)

In these lines, a hyperawareness of the boundaries of Black lifestyles mingles the Black oral-urban vernacular with modernist concretism, to drive home the futility of deluded human desires in a racist world. Turning racial restrictions into boundaries that positively define Black life, Lee warns against temptations to "forget" and "wander as I wonder" in a race-free reverie. As the Muslim rejects pork to strengthen his identity, the Black person, by refusing to transgress, controls the "nevers" in his world.

In a more playful mode, Lee's "communication in whi-te" is a satirical verbivocovisual text that assaults the reader's eyes with its clusters of "e's," "g's," "l's." The rapid sounds aurally match the sound of automatic weapons, and onomatopoiecally the poem embodies the sense of the Vietnam War that the Paris Peace talks failed to solve. Just as the Peace talks seemed rooted in a lack of integrity, coherence, and control, the typography slips from one word into another. In perhaps the most clever line of the poem, the sound of guns ("te te") slides into the French word for a close meeting, i.e., "tete-a-tete," which of course here is satirical, a good example of Lee's biting wit:

> communication in whi-te
>
> dee dee dee dee dee wee weee eeeeee wee we
>   deweeeeeeee ee ee ee nig
> nig nig nig niggggggggggggggggggg cleek cleek cleek
>   cleeeeee cleekcleek
> rip rip rip rip rip/rip/rip/rip/rip/ripripripripripripripri
>   pi pi pi pi pip
> bom bom bom bom bom/bom/bom/bombombombom
>   bombbombbombbombbombbomb
> deathtocleekdeathtocleekdeathtocleekdeathtocleek
>   deathtocleekdeathtodeathto
> allllllllllllallllllllllll alllllllllll deathtoalllllllll alllllllll
>   alllllllleeeeeeee
> te te te te te te te/te/te/te/te/te/tetetetetetetetetete
>   tetetetetetete:
> the paris peace talks, 1968.
> (*Don't Cry, Scream*, p. 23)

As in Rodgers' poem, Don L. Lee's typography and orthography seem deeply integrated in his craft and coordinated to carry his ideas, even in his prose. For instance, in the introduction to his third chapbook, *Don't Cry, Scream* (1969), the fulsome list of names of persons who helped him develop as a poet appears in a solid block of text, without upper case letters or punctuation. The

effect is to suggest a solid "foundation" of mentors and to underscore their "communality." Following this tribute, Lee signs his
own name with a minimalist, "dll," suggesting, perhaps, his own
modest role as a black everyman poet. Finally he explains the
origin of his title as advice from his mother (who died at age
thirty-five in a Detroit ghetto when Lee was a teenager). Lee
explains, with suitable visual effect, that his mother's advice was,
"if u is goin to open yr/mouth DON'T CRY, SCREAM." Here,
without equivocation, Lee expresses his awareness that language
must be manipulated on several planes.

If critics found such uses of altered type pretentious such criticism generally overlooked the possibility of a Black visual poetics,
imperfect at times, but serious in its efforts. Only recently, in the
Nommo anniversary volume, has a critic, himself an OBAC poet,
attempted serious analysis of the visual craft of another Black
Chicago poet. D. L. Crockett-Smith notes the role of spacing,
altered lines and spelling in the work of OBAC poet Angela
Jackson in his essay, "Angela Jackson."[12] While Crockett finds
some of Jackson's experiments arbitrary and less than effective, on
the whole he applauds her creative craft. In the final analysis,
however, he links her visual spacing and unorthodox spelling
closer to the aurality of her work than to its visual structure.

Besides Rodgers' and Lee's early publications, the Chicago
poets' stress on the visual side of poetry is amply represented in an
anthology dedicated to Gwendolyn Brooks entitled *To Gwen With
Love*. Published in 1971 by the Johnson Publishing Company of
Chicago, *To Gwen* epitomizes the communal and creative spirit of
the Chicago Black Arts movement. Yet, despite its social and
ideological context, the poetry in *To Gwen* shows persistent en-
gagement with questions of poetic process, particularly questions
that involve the materiality of words. Of the fifty-four represented
poets, the majority show strong stress on the visual side of poetry,
with varying degrees of interest in the oral aspect. Most clearly,
however, these sociopoets combine modernist concretism with
their project of reflecting conceptual and ideological "truths." That
in so doing they were in a sense still heirs of Black modern-

ists can be seen when two poems are compared. These two poems, the much anthologized "We Real Cool"[13] by Gwendolyn Brooks and "Gwen Brooks, A Pyramid"[14] by the actress/poet Val Gray Ward, illustrate in microcosm the continuity and change from Black modernism to the Black Arts aesthetic. They also illustrate a change in cultural climate from social protest to cultural affirmation. But formally, they show the movement from a subordinate visual aesthetic to a predominant visual aesthetic.

To begin with, as with Herbert and Rodgers' poems discussed above, both poems present the shape of a pyramid, Brooks' being an inverted pyramid and Ward's upright. Here are the texts:

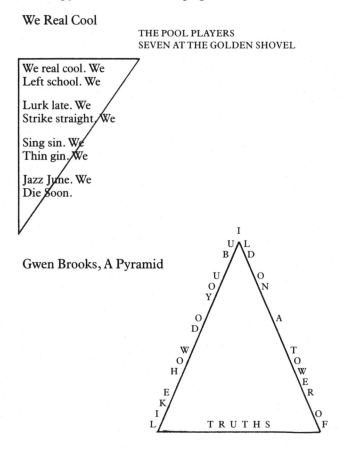

We Real Cool

THE POOL PLAYERS
SEVEN AT THE GOLDEN SHOVEL

We real cool. We
Left school. We

Lurk late. We
Strike straight. We

Sing sin. We
Thin gin. We

Jazz June. We
Die soon.

Gwen Brooks, A Pyramid

As an inverted pyramid Brook's poem's visual pattern turns the meaning of this icon upside down. The pyramid, an icon used on American currency, conventionally represents strength and stability. Yet here the longest of a series of short lines occurs at the top of the poem, and the shortest line, recalling Herbert's "with thee/ Most poor," occurs at the poem's end, suggesting, as in Herbert's inverted pyramid, decline, diminution, and death. But here there is no hope of rebirth, no spreading line following after to suggest either stability or escape on wings of spiritual flight. Published in her "most social" (i.e., racially protesting) volume, "We Real Cool" seems to be a poem only about death in the city and wasted lives. Here wisdom is folly, social order is threatened by the lumpenproletariat, and history succumbs to a fatal ignorance. The patterns of "We's" at the end of each line follow this interpretation, suggesting the open endedness of indecision and foolish bravado, while the breathlessness of the vowel suggests the danger signal of a blown whistle ("weeee"), screaming emergency/urgency, and cautionary restraint, even as the boys rush to their decline.

On a visual level, the pattern of "We's" presents a problem because they seem to disrupt the pyramid underlying the verbal text. Once the series of declarative statements is established, the "We's" stray further and further from the inverted apex of the pyramid. If, at first, this observation invites denial of the role of a visual graph underlying the poem's discourse, however, interpretation of such "deviance" is equally inviting. The "We's" may suggest multivocality, for instance. The boys' group voice in the first person of the first three or four sentences may be separated from a later first person plural that includes the implied author and her audience. Thus, in a sense, Brooks offers two versions of transgression in "We Real Cool." On one hand, the boys transgress social and moral codes: they have left school; they defy curfews, they like bad things; they not only drink gin but corrupt it; they waste the "summers" of their lives; and although Brooks has denied it during her readings of the poems, they may be guilty of gang rape ("Jazz June"). Finally, in defiance of nature's law that death is for the old, these adolescents "die soon." In the end, however, Brooks transgresses her own modernist code of aesthetic self-sufficiency if the final "We's" are seen as deliberate disruptions of the text. Given the urgency of the social crisis, more important than a perfectly crafted text is the impulse to step "outside" the paradigm of defeat and issue a command call-and-response challenge.

"We Real Cool" thus reveals Brooks' manipulation of and interest in spatialism (as many of her titles and frequent epigrams also indicate)[15] as a way to underscore her message. As one critic noted about European and American visual poetry in general, this kind of aesthetic indicates a commitment to wholistic art, to "symbiosis of organic structures that affect each other to advantage: . . . not a logical but a ubicentric poetry, a multiple textual space that implies the gesture as its context."[16]

Turning to Ward's poem, because its meaning is inseparable from its shape, it is more closely allied to the graphic and plastic arts than Brooks' poem. Visually and ideologically, the poem offers an alternative not only to the pyramid as it is presented in conventional American iconology, i.e., on the American dollar where its seems aligned with a capitalist exchange ethos, but also to the negative inverted pyramid in Rodgers' and Brooks' poems cited earlier. Here the pyramid, as an icon of Egyptian culture, would be meant to represent an image of Africanity – African wisdom, aristocracy, historicity, stability, foundations, and culture. Interestingly, the placing of the letter "i" at the top of the pyramid forms a visual pun, suggesting simultaneously the personal pronoun "I" and the "eye" as an organ of physical sight and insight (wisdom). Unlike pure abstract concrete poetry, the personalism of this poem and its accessible message prevent the poem from being a simple obscure "modernist" exercise in the manipulation of letters. Here concretism carries a didactic discourse and the image becomes interrogative, presenting discourse as the figure and the figure as discourse, co-expressing being and dialogism simultaneously. If Brooks sounded an alarm, Ward issues a challenge, playing on the call and response convention of Afro-American vernacular culture. Like the pentecostal preacher, Ward is asking, albeit visually, "Can I get a witness?"

From the above observations it should be apparent that the Chicago Black Arts poets were neither purely provincial nor racial in their aesthetic impulse. Rather, they participated in a counter-culture aesthetic both local and international in scope, reaching back to Mallarmé, the Dadaists, and even to the religious poets of the seventeenth century while encompassing their urban culture. Like their European and American counterparts they were attempting to humanize and expand print, to riff on the typewriter, to reach their roots in gesture, incantation, and ritual; to unite eye, ear, and body in dance, voice, and glance. They wanted to recover themselves as communal and social persons, freed from usurptive cultural boundaries. In their quest for a visual aesthetic, Lee, Rodgers, Ward, and other OBAC poets pushed writing past illusionism to a concretist mimesis that altered language and the reading process and at the same time revealed the limitations of both.

Notes

[1] Quoted in Michel Fabre, "Langston Hughes' Literary Reputation in France," *The Langston Hughes Review* (Spring, 1987), p. 25.

[2] Quoted from the poem, "Black Art," in Dudley Randall, ed., *The Black Poets* (New York: Bantam Books, 1971), p. 224.

[3] Most of my background information on the OBAC has been taken from Carole A. Parks, ed., *NOMMO: A Literary Legacy of Black Chicago (1967-1987)* (Chicago: OBAhouse, 1987). This anniversary anthology contains poetry and essays by over 50 past and current OBAC members. A look at the credits shows that the five writers cited have published over thirty volumes. Cited in the text as *NOMMO*.

[4] Hoyt W. Fuller's "Foreword" to the 1971 issue of OBAC's journal, *NOMMO*.

[5] David Antin, "Modernism and Postmodernism: Approaching the Present in American Poetry," in Richard Kostelanetz, ed., *The Avant-garde Tradition in Literature* (New York: Prometheus Books, 1982), pp. 216-247.

[6] Don L. Lee, "The Black Christ," *Black Pride* (Detroit, 1968), p. 22.

[7] Don L. Lee, "Black Writing," in Gwendolyn Brooks, ed., *Jump Bad: A New Chicago Anthology* (Detroit: Broadside Press, 1971) pp. 37-39. Cited in the text as *Jump Bad*. In about 1972, Don L. Lee changed his name to Haki Madhubuti, but

when he published his three signal chapbooks it was as Lee; therefore I will retain this usage.

⁸ Carolyn Rodgers, "The Literature of Black," in *Black World* (June, 1970), p. 10. Cited in the text as Rodgers.

⁹ Among the core texts for this climactic period from 1968 to about 1972, are Don L. Lee's *Think Black!* (Detroit: Broadside Press, 1967), *Black Pride* (Detroit: Broadside Press, 1968), and *Don't Cry, Scream* (Detroit: Broadside Press, 1969); Rodgers' *Paper Soul* (Chicago: Third World Press, 1968) and *Songs of a Blackbird* (Chicago: Third World Press, 1969); Gwendolyn Brooks' anthology *Jump Bad* (cited above), and Patricia L. Brown, Don L. Lee, and Francis Ward, eds., *To Gwen with Love: An Anthology Dedicated to Gwendolyn Brooks* (Chicago: Johnson Publishing, 1971). A host of other poets self-published chapbooks or published in journals emanating from places other than Chicago. They will be studied in future essays. Also crucial locally was Fuller's position as managing editor of John H. Johnson's *Negro Digest* (renamed *Black World* in 1970). For more information on Fuller's influence see the section, "Remembering Hoyt W. Fuller," in *NOMMO* (1987), pp. 293-335.

¹⁰ George Herbert, "Easter Wings," in X. J. Kennedy, ed., *An Introduction To Poetry* (Boston: Little, Brown, 1986), p. 193.

¹¹ For an example of Rodgers' use of innovative spelling and "Black English" in prose, see her essay, "Black Poetry – Where It's At," reprinted in *NOMMO* (1987), pp. 28-37. Rodgers seems to link her usage here more clearly to the sound of black speech. She writes about *teachin, rappin,* and *bein* poems, for example, using the lost "g's" to reflect lost consonants in so-called characteristic black vernacular speech. My emphasis here is on the *visual* impact of altered spelling, only incidentally on altered spelling that is used to suggest *oral* speech patterns.

¹² David L. Crockett Smith, "Angela Jackson," in *NOMMO*, pp. 38-44.

¹³ Gwendolyn Brooks, "We Real Cool," in the *World of Gwendolyn Brooks* (New York: Harper and Row, 1971), p, 331.

¹⁴ Val Gray Ward, "Gwen Brooks, A Pyramid," in Patricia L. Brown, Don L. Lee, and Francis Ward, eds. *To Gwen with Love: An Anthology Dedicated to Gwendolyn Brooks* (Chicago: Johnson Publishing, 1971), p. 99.

¹⁵ See my essay on Brooks' use of collage spatial techniques in her war sonnets in "The Step of Iron Feet: Creative Practice in the War Sonnets of Melvin B. Tolson and Gwendolyn Brooks," *Obsidian II: Black Literature in Review*, 2 (Winter, 1987), 69-87.

¹⁶ Paul de Vree, "Visual Poetry," in Kostelánetz, ed., *The Avant-Garde Tradition in Literature*, p. 347.

Transplanting Roots and Taking Off: Latino Poetry in Illinois*

Marc Zimmerman

University of Illinois at Chicago

Backgrounds

Where are the latin poets?
Maybe at the neighborhood tavern,
    like the
rest of the latins drowning their thoughts
on American beer or wine.
Thinking about back home
where the land is warm.
Yes, thinking about mi viejita.

Wine is fine when the mind unwinds
thoughts such as, why?
Sleeping in the snow when our
    country
is so warm,
where are the latin poets?
I don't know, maybe sleeping in
    the snow
or vacationing down at Cook
    County Jail.[1]

B Y VIRTUE of its content as well as by its strategic appearance in two key Chicago-area Latino publications in the late 1970s, this poem by a young Chicago Rican raises and also begins to answer the questions which must concern us in this first effort to trace the history of Illinois Latino poetry. As midwestern and Illinois poetry developed in relation to national trends, what was happening with respect to midwest Latino literature and poetry? The national Latino population had expanded; and by the 1960s, a number of young Chicano and Puerto Rican writers had emerged. They had begun to forge new literary forms, characterized by nostalgia for a fading past; by a critique of racial oppression and negative acculturation experiences in the fields, the city neighborhoods, the schools, factories, and homes; by bilingualisms, schizophrenic goal conflicts, and sex role confusions; by

---

*This study is based on Part I of a book-in-progress on Illinois Latino poetry. I wish to acknowledge the invaluable participation of Carlos Cumpián of *MARCH, INC.*, Movimiento Artistico Chicano, who serves as archivist, critic, and constant interlocutor for the work-in-progress.

77

cultural tensions, affirmations, and anger; and by calls for reform, rebellion, revolution, or other forms of opposition. These new literary forms attempted to serve as laboratories for the expression and then reconstruction of transformed Latin American and U.S. Southwest Hispano-Indian peoples into "Mexican-Americans" or "Chicanos," into "Nuyorikans" or other Ricans, and ultimately, into the conglomerate we know today as "Hispanics" or (the word preferred in Chicago) "Latinos."

Of course, few people knew of the literary work emerging among the chicanos and boricuas. Professional writers and critics (non-Latinos almost all) were slow to recognize and come to respect even their greatest early achievements. It was common for budding Latino writers in different parts of the U.S. to be unaware of the existence of other Latino writers; and even when burgeoning Chicano and Puerto Rican literary movements had emerged in relation to growing Latino national consciousness and action, few Latinos living in the U.S. were aware of the literature. But what could one expect when millions of Latinos only had limited functional literacy in Spanish or English and when most Latinos were consigned to blue-collar or no-collar jobs, if they found work at all? It took the first relatively large-scale wave of Latino students in U.S. universities, in the context of the civil rights movement and the emergence of an anti-establishment, anti-Vietnam War counter culture, to produce both the writers and readers of this new literature.

In the Midwest, and Illinois, where the Latino population and Latino cultural nationalism had developed slower than in the Southwest or the East Coast, more slowly, the process by which Latino literary expression developed was even slower. More cut off from prior rural roots and traditions, midwestern and more specifically Illinois Latino literature would be somewhat different from the national norm; and just as midwestern Latinos were slower to register as part of the national Latino totality, so would be those who expressed Latino concerns through literature.

Latino literature would develop, however, though it would not do so primarily as a phenomenon rooted in Illinois or the Midwest, and not as something tied closely to the general characteristics of the region, but as a phenomenon tied to a great urb, to that great center of immigration and immigrant literature: Chicago. Where were Illinois's Latin poets? Well, there were a few here and there in migrant and university centers around the state. But, in the main, they were in the city, for the city connected them with a movement which fed their development. They were in the city, in its enclaves, barrios, and schools, in all the real and metaphorical jails and refuges provided for those marginalized by forlorn and inhospitable urban circumstances. Of course some of them who could free themselves and grow actually found a way through the maze of bilingualisms and biculturalisms to express themselves in written words. Some of these even found their way into the few publications that would publish their work – or into the new publications they or friends created which served as outlets they otherwise had great difficulty finding, either nationally, or in Chicago itself.

Mexican and then Mexican texano immigration to the Midwest and Illinois began early in the 20th century, during the Mexican Revolution, in relation to the demand for labor on the railroads, in field work, and of course in the steel mills and meatpacking plants. Through ups and downs, periods of mass deportations, and expanding immigration, that population base continued to expand, and to be joined after World War II by a major Puerto Rican exodus, principally to Chicago. Obviously 1959 and 1980 marked the key dates of two major and very different Cuban migrations. In between, large numbers came from Ecuador, Colombia, Chile, and elsewhere. After 1980, numerous Guatemalans and Salvadorans have added to a population base which continues to expand because of high birth rates in the U.S. and economic crisis in Mexico.

By the late 1960s, both major immigration waves into the Midwest were well established. And now a new, more articulate generation had come forth to voice and seek solutions to a series of unresolved and deepening problems facing the groups. To be sure, national Latino political activism in New York, California, and Texas influenced Illinois developments, but the state, and above all Chicago, was to make its own unique contribution. The same was to be true in the related area of cultural and literary developments in which the socio-economic and political problems and possible solutions would be projected and expressed.

The Mexican and Puerto Rican migrations to the U.S. were primarily workingclass in nature, and the groups brought with them those elements of their national and Latin American culture, oral tradition, and literature available to their social class and situations. For a distinct U.S. Latino culture and literature to emerge for each group, there had to be sufficient experience of U.S. life, culture, and language to pressure Latin American cultural norms, and there had to be a sufficient degree of critical consciousness, generated through hardship, but articulated through institutional or extra-institutional / counter-cultural formations to make writing as a vehicle of cultural definition both necessary and possible. Obviously that literary expression required an adequate pooling of resources for at least minimal cultural reproduction and distribution – from self-publishing to small chapbook and literary journal production. To the degree that the emergent literatures tended to stand in relation to broader cultural and socio-psychological patterns, they tended to parallel developments elsewhere, but they were marked by certain characteristics specific to the Midwest and especially to its prime urb, Chicago.

Clearly the resources available would affect literary production, as would the specific characteristics of Latino populations in given areas. But U.S. Latino literary development might be loosely divided into three phases. The first phase is a romantic literature attempting to replicate the homebase literary culture with variations in subjects, emphases, and expressive modes deriving from the particularities of the writer's origins and experience. This usually means a nostalgic, nationalistic poetry of loss and exile, rhymed, romantic, rhetorical, and declamatory in style with conventional rhythms, rhyming patterns, and poetic techniques. Mexican corridos, Puerto Rican plenas, and other musical forms influenced this literary expression, as did folklore, sayings, proverbs, etc. It is male-centered, affirms tradition and traditional sex roles, sees change as loss and decadence.

The second phase is a literature of immigration, marked by hopes, but also by problems, presenting everyday confusions and conflicts, etc., and frequently exploring racism and national identity, affirming roots, appealing to justice, and envisioning social solutions. This literature is primarily in song and poetry, but it is also in fictional and dramatic form. It is a literature only somewhat mediated by existing literary norms. It is performative, social, didactic, hortatory; it is often bitter, militant, defiant. Still close to oral roots, it may play far better than it reads. It's meant to be read and heard by targeted groups in specific settings. In poetry, this is a literature without rhyme, jagged in rhythm, imitating emergent musical forms, with some influences based on conceptions of Black or American Indian cultures. Still male and tradition-centered, these positions begin to be undermined by more critical perspectives. Change through immigration and acculturation leads to new syntheses, some of which are seen as creative.

The third phase is a literature of settlement, also looking back on the homebase and immigration, but from a more settled-in framework, with an existing Latino tradition behind it, now reaching out to other minority and mainstream traditions (U.S. mainly but also Latin American, African, etc.). It was an attempt to expand horizons and move either to pan-Latin American, "pan-third world," or U.S. mainstream identifications. Here the culture itself becomes increasingly self-critical; feminist and post-nationalist issues become central, as do a wide range of alternative cultural models and directions. Expression is frequently more individual, subjective, inward; style replaces a generalized rhetoric. In one sense this literature may be an expression of assimilation or acculturation that may or may not represent the broader group aggregate (but rather a sector thereof), but it may also be a literature which draws upon, even as it critically distances itself from, earlier norms and suppositions.

These phases are far from exclusive. Tendencies exist along a continuum. Midwestern and specifically Illinois-Chicago Latino literature developed late when U.S. Latino consciousness and literature was moving along the continuum from the second to the

third phase. An assumption in what follows is that Chicago and
more broadly Illinois Latino literature telescopes the second and
third phases to produce a literature which still has roots in the
barrio, but which tends to project beyond national to broader
Latino and universal concerns.

The fact is, Latino poetry and literature existed in the Midwest
and in Chicago since the earliest Mexicans came to the area.
Adaptations and transformations of corridos and poems from the
declamatory school of Mexican poetry could be heard in bars, and
were occasionally published in some of the early Latino newspapers and journals. The first masterpiece of Chicano fiction, Texas-
born Tomás Rivera's *no se lo trag la tierra* (*And the Earth Did not
Devour Him*, 1972), has episodes in the fields of Iowa and Minnesota, and bespeaks the presence of deep *tejano* traditions extending throughout the Midwest along the trails of migrant farmwork.
More germane to our subject, the most important early Chicano
poet of Chicago, Carlos Cortez, was born and raised in Milwaukee,
one of the main midwestern urbs to which railroading Mexican
and settled-out Texas migrants gravitated in their search for new
industrial jobs. But while there are Latino-oriented works among
Cortez's earliest poems, he was not writing in a strict Latino
framework, or as part of an existent Latino circuit. He would in
fact participate in the emergence of that framework and circuit in
the late 60s and early 70s. But it is not until 1971 that Latino
writing would have its first organized spurt and there would be
consistent development leading to the turning point years of
1976-79.

A specifically U.S. Latino ethnic literature emerged in Chicago
as the Latino population and its problems grew in the explosive
climate of the late 1960s, which found its most overt expression in
the Black and Puerto Rican riots of 1967 and the 1968 Democratic
Convention riots. Minority and poverty problems led to new programs and new resources; social service centers started cultural
programs; culture was considered as part of the answer to the
general social question. Various "cultural workers" and "modes of
cultural production" emerged: folk singers, street and stage per-

formers, visual artists, essayists, poets, theater groups, writers' workshops, – and, yes, new publications.

The Chicago-based publication, *The Rican: A Journal of Contemporary Puerto Rican Thought*, edited by Samuel Betances, appeared in 1971 and published important pieces (including poems) on Puerto Rican identity until its demise in 1975; chapbooks by Puerto Rican David Hernández and Chicano Carlos Morton also appeared in 1971. The next year, at the University of Indiana Northwest, in Gary, another Puerto Rican, Nicolás Kanellos, founded *Revista Chicano-Riqueña* which became the major national publication bringing together key Chicano and Puerto Rican writers (including several from Chicago). Also in 1972 the organization MARCH, Inc. (Movimiento Artistico Chicano) was founded in Hammond, Indiana, to promote Chicano visual arts; and by mid 1976, MARCH started publishing their arts and poetry journal, *Abrazo*. Then in 1977, the *Revista Chicano-Riqueña* published its special Chicago issue, *Nosotros: A Collection of Latino Poetry and Graphics from Chicago*, which offered the first focused presentation of Chicago-based Latino cultural production and first called national attention to a virtual Latino emergence in the Chicago area. At roughly the same time, Carlos Heredia began promoting Southside Mexicano writing, publishing some issues of a journal called *Imagines* and founding Alternativa Press to publish the first chapbook of Ana Castillo. In 1978, Marilou Castillo produced a book of poetry; in 1979, *Abrazo* appeared for a second and final issue; *Revista Chicano-Riqueña* left Gary, Indiana, for bigger and better things at the University of Houston, eventually changing its name to *Américas Review*; and a small journal, *Ecos*, based at the University of Illinois at Chicago, made a modest effort to fill the local void. In 1980, at the University of Indiana in Bloomington, Norma Alarcón established a new major vehicle for Illinois Latina writers, *Third Woman*, and a new Chicago Chicana writer, Sandra Cisneros, produced her first chapbook. A new stage of Latino literature was in the offing.

When we discuss Illinois Latino literature, then, we are referring to an arc of roughly twenty years, from the late 60s to the present.

At the center of this arc is the period from the mid to late 1970s, which was marked by the two publications which best summarize the past and point toward the future: the *Revista Chicano-Riqueña* (especially the issue entitled *Nosotros*), and *Abrazo*. Matías's "Where are the Latin Poets?" appeared first in *Nosotros*, and was then re-published in the second issue of *Abrazo* (1979). So much happened throughout the 1960s and 70s, so many new Chicago Latino poets emerged, that the question raised in his simple little poem was already being answered; the contents and orientation of the poem, its dual appearance and the publications in which it appeared, sum up a good deal of what was at stake.

Even though very few still knew about it, Illinois "Latin" or rather "Latino" poets had arrived and were taking root; and now they were proclaiming their advent with public performances and publications. In the deepest sense, for Matías, all Latinos, like all humans, were poets, but they were poets with a special problem, caught between two places and two languages. In effect, they were poets who had no easy means to express themselves, and who were cut off from most of Latin American literary traditions. It is only today that some of the emerging university-trained Latino writers are in a position to make contact with the great élite Latin American literary tradition, whose class and linguistic roots within the Hispanic domain are not the same as the roots for the U.S. writers.

The Latino poets were trapped in a cold urban reality, nostalgic for a rural or smalltown past they romanticized in memory and fantasy, and sometimes traumatized, marginalized, dazed, and jailed as a result of their experience. What could they write to free themselves and others from their "mind jails"? What could they do but reproduce the sights and sounds they knew – the street language of their people attempting to survive and thrive in the midst of a society fraught with difficulty and danger? So it was to be, for Matías and his contemporaries in Chicago. Building on national and local social, cultural, and literary developments, they would create a new urban poetry, with glances back at the *tierra natal*, but mainly with a look to how they and the thousands of voiceless poets they hoped to represent might find expression and new life. They also sought to reach beyond the Chicago jail-world, and sometimes even their ethnic collectivity, to speak of history, individual problems, the cosmos. But the first question about them was: would they be able to say things of importance to and about their immediate world? Would they be able to make ideological and aesthetic contributions to their peoples, the area, state, and region in which they lived?

A final, not insignificant point to note in this context is that although eight of the ten poets collected in the *Nosotros* issue were Puerto Rican, and while *Abrazo* was the product of a group designated as "Chicano," the poets referred to by Matías are "Latin" – not Puerto Rican or Chicano. Here we are at the very center of things important to Chicago's Latino world and its poets. Both publications pointed to the significant links between Chicago Latino poetry and other arts, between art and culture and broader community concerns. Both publications, while products of local efforts, implicitly and explicitly linked Chicago Latinos to the Latino past, present, and future in U.S. and hemispheric terms. Both, in spite of their particular nationalist priorities, involved creators from the two prime groups constituting Chicago's Latino community and the national Latino community as well. Indeed, both publications performed that task which was implicit in the very name of the *Revista Chicano-Riqueña* and which would constitute perhaps the major contribution of Chicago to the Latino totality in Illinois, the Midwest, and the nation: an extension beyond given national consciousness to a more general Hispanic or Latino consciousness as a step in articulating group concerns necessary for political and social dialogue and struggle.[2]

If up to the time of these publications, few people had heard much about "Chicago Hispanic poets" or even "Chicago Hispanics," now Chicago *Latinismo* was to come of age with a newly heightened Latino definition and thrust. *Nosotros* is crucial to our story because it brought together poets in a nationally distributed Latino journal and because it highlighted Puerto Rican talent in a city which in terms of things Latino, was mainly seen as Mexican. While *Revista* had carried some Chicago poets and artists from its early days, with its *Nosotros* issue featuring ten Latino poets and several visual artists, Chicago Latino poetry and art were finally on the national map.

Above all, *Nosotros* specifically and consciously articulated Chicago's pan-nationalist Latino perspective, using the militant language of the times but nevertheless summing up issues which remain crucial to this day:

> We are the Latino poets and artists. As Boricuas and Chicanos we have struggled to define ourselves and erase the stereotypes imposed on our minds by the forces of oppression. The Latino communities of America have said, "Basta/Enough!" No longer will Latinos in the U.S.A. be identified and stereotyped with images of what Puerto Ricans, Cubans, Mexicans should act like as seen through the eyes of the world. We will identify ourselves. We will decide who we are and what we will be about. We exercise the right to express our identity so that no exploiter could confuse and use us. . . . Our poetry and art is born of love, of suffering, and of every experience that delights and torments our people. We are the magicians who weave glorious spells of thought images, depicting the lives, moods, struggles, and hopes of the people who populate the Latino barrios of Chicago. We print rainbows of thoughts and feelings that range from the darkest hues of anger and bitterness to the brightest fantasies and dreams. . . . We speak with the voices of a rainbow underground that is beginning to surface from the pitfalls of racism; for we will not eliminate but harmonize our Afro-Indio-Hispano roots and our children of every color will set an example of brotherhood to all mankind.[3]

Where did the *Nosotros* poets come from and where were they going? In what way were they typical of their moment, or at least the Chicago Puerto Rican experience at that time? To what degree do they culminate past developments and anticipate the future? As a frame for exploring Illinois Latino poetry, we should examine the work of the key *Nosotros* poet, David Hernández, as a means for showing how the social and literary past of Chicago and Illinois Latino poets leads not just to nationalism, but to perspectives which move beyond it to a vision of *latinidad*, and then still further towards internationalism as well as the possibility of a future multi-racial rainbow coalition. A look at Hernández will give us an encapsulized view of the story of Puerto Rican literature in Chicago. We will then give an extended treatment of the Mexican/ Chicano story flowing into and out of *Abrazo*, to see how those two stories lead to others both in Chicago and in the state as a whole.

Early Chicago Rican Poets and David Hernández

Puerto Rican poetry written in Chicago exists prior to the major settlement wave, with the first Puerto Ricans to come to the area. It now seems clear that there are *plenas*, poems of nostalgia and exile, written in Chicago long before the 1970s which must be found, collected, and examined if the whole story of Chicago Rican poetry is to be told. However, for our purposes, the situation which most specifically leads to the emergence of a Puerto Rican literature in Chicago stems from the conditions of economic and social marginalization and alienation which produced the Puerto Rican Division Street riot of 1967 and led to the formation of new organizations and groups attempting to generate more positive developments in the Puerto Rican Community. Just as ABC, Aspira, Inc., and other community organizations developed, so did high school, university, and community centers and groups, which saw cultural expression as at least one dimension of their work. The emergence of collective publication projects is clearly part of this story.[4]

From 1971 until its demise in 1975, Samuel Betances' Chicago-based publication, *The Rican: A Journal of Puerto Rican Cultural Expression*, was to produce many seminal articles on questions of Puerto Rican island and immigration history and experience, and usually included at least some poems, primarily those written by young Chicago Puerto Ricans. Some of these poets were also involved in the new social organizations (Carmelo Rodrguez would come to head ASPIRA); some would become members of community arts organizations such as *El Taller* (The Workshop) and ALBA and would also be among the *Nosotros* writers. In this latter category were David Hernández, Julio Noboa, Carmelo Romero, and Emma Iris Rodrguez; but Chico Rivera and Shabazz Prez were other young Puerto Ricans who wrote poetry for the journal.

Some of these writers, and above all Hernández, would be among the first Chicago Latino writers to appear in the pages of *Revista Chicano-Riqueña*. But clearly, the key early continuity was between the poets of *The Rican* who found their way, through the *Nosotros* collective, into *Revista Chicano-Riqueña*'s *Nosotros* issue. The central figure in the *Nosotros* group, the writer who encouraged many of them and served as their mentor and model, was David Hernández, who has figured as a major personality and poet in the Chicago/Illinois Latino scene to this day.

For most non-Latino Chicagoans who know anything about Latino poetry, Hernández *is* Chicago Latino poetry. He's the perennial ubiquitous representative, the one let in the front door, the talented "token" in citywide, statewide, nationwide anthologies, our Nuyorican poet Chi-town style.[5] Of course for some Latinos and Puerto Ricans, he remains too disreputable, too connected with bohemianism, drugs, booze, jazz, black culture, white culture. He's too much a paradox: at once the Chicago institution and alternative model for young Rican gangbangers; yet too anarchistic, too anti-establishment, too beat, hippie, and the rest. Some complain about his unwillingness to join a specific Puerto Rican political group, even as he works for and is identified with the most progressive political trends in Chicago. Some complain he takes Puerto Rican problems too lightly. But the fact is that Hernández has taken on the traditional stance of the poet manqué. Whether in truth or in fantasy, he has taken on the persona of a Puerto Rican Whitman or Hart Crane, singing fiercely democratic and populist hymns to the bums, drunks, losers, and bag ladies, all those whose fates are somehow likenable to the worst things possible in the Puerto Rican diaspora.

The fact also is that by means of his chimerical poetic identity, he has been able to stand for many of the identity possibilities and directions that exist in the Puerto Rican community. He has had, then, the "negative capability" Keats ascribed to a fairly well-known poet, and which has enabled Hernández to represent many – the men if not all the women. Hernández has sought to be Chicago's complete Puerto Rican male voice, has sought to express the entire range of pre-feminist U.S. Puerto Rican literary themes, from nostalgia over roots, to growing up Latino in the rough part of town, to the struggle to win equality and recognition, to an expansion beyond the Puerto Rican and more broadly Latino world to the still larger world beyond. This gamut is present in Hernández's collection in 1971, significantly called *Despertando* (*Waking Up*).[6]

As far as we can gather, *Despertando* is the first poetry collection by a Chicago Latino. Not fortuitously, it appeared in the same year that *The Rican* was born, and on the eve of the birth of *Revista Chicano-Riqueña*. The title is derived from the nationalist chant, *Despierta Boricua, defiende lo tuyo* (*Wake up Puerto Ricans, defend what's yours*). The refrain was constantly heard in Chicago's Puerto Rican neighborhoods, especially in the 1970s. It is present as well in the poems which appear in the *Nosotros* issue and in Hernández's later work. The volume itself is very uneven (almost all the best, most realized poems are in the first pages of the book); and in this way, it anticipates not only most of Hernández's themes but also his main characteristics as a writer. Here, with the question of unevenness, we should be a bit careful, however. For, as his first book shows, Hernández's art situates itself as a virtual manifesto of creative improvisation.

Capable of rewriting and rewriting a given poem year after year, Hernández nevertheless insists, through form and overt statement, on the crucial, inviolable status of inspiration and spontaneity. Since part of his art is an irreverence to academic poetics, his trick is frequently to create a poem which seems unpremeditated and unchecked, even when the effect may prove ultimately calculated. The poems are written as variants of an unstated melody or set of chords, in function of a given rhythm design, with internal rhymes and other poetic baggage creating a sense of form which is then continually violated, usually in a gentle and mocking way, as if the dissonance or rhythmic interruption is a function of life's or society's confusions, disequilibria, and discord. Since 1972, Hernández has usually read his poems with his musical group, *los Sonidos de la Calle* or Street Sounds (currently bass, guitar, congas, and other percussion in a Latin-jazz synchretism that parallels and complements the mixing process found in the poems themselves). And since the Sounds supply the unheard undercurrent music and rhythm, the full effect of Hernández's stylistic tricks come to the fore; as the half-shaped, purposely offbeat line plays out against the more truly formed notes and chord patterns, the dissonance, interruptedness, and tentativeness of one between two cultural systems, belief patterns, and imperatives emerge. Perhaps this is Hernández's challenge as a writer: many of his poems don't work as well on paper as they do against a musical background. Part of this question is one of personality, but in the 1980s, theatrical productions based on his poems have proven them effective even when he was not directly delivering them.

The references to music and theater are just indications of the broad artistic orientations sometimes hidden by Hernández's populist thematics and attitudes. So, when asked about his inspiration, his reference is not to music or theater but to sculpture.[7] "Poetry is the tool to change the English language," he says.

> I am out to destroy the language of silly fascists and rebuild it for all of us. This white sculptor Julian Harr took me into his studio in 1963 and I became his apprentice. Not as a sculptor but as a poet. Watching him carve and chip away, create form out of formlessness is how I learned the craft of poetry. My life was half into my people and half into the artist counter-cultural bohemian life-style that Julian represented. From there on my circle of artists from all races and backgrounds grew larger until all hell broke loose and I found my heaven.

But after this trip into sculpture, the reference seems to go into music after all: "I am a product of the African Griot, and the antenna of the race. Poetry is important to me because it fills the space between my heart-beats."

Born in Cidra, Puerto Rico, in 1946, Hernández arrived in Chicago with his parents, two brothers, and a sister in 1955. As one of his more recent poems tells us, his parents were very poor. They lived mainly on the Puerto Rican northside, and he went to three different grade schools – demoted, displaced, and spewed through and out of the educational system "because no spik English."

In the late 60s, he was already a member of the counter-culture, into drugs, jazz, and (if we can believe his poetry) lots of hetero-sex. Dedicating his work to all those whom he can call his people and community, his poems tumbled out, half hacked, half formed, bits and pieces taken here and there, some impressions on Chicago's CTA, vignettes out of Chicago night lights, some personal remembrances which, taken together, might make a little novel, a miniature version of a Latino life, like Eduardo Rivera's *Family Installments*, or a male version of Sandra Cisneros' *House on Mango Street*. So, *Despertando* starts in Puerto Rico with a boy climbing up a mountain, tin pail full, dogs barking and singing behind him. Next he is on a plane, arriving at Midway. A proud boy but brown, anticipating the smiles of Americans, he arrives and is hit by the Chicago wind. And as the book unfolds, we see him get to know his new world. There are poems about Puerto Ricans young and old, about lumpens brown, black and white. There's a Puerto Rican man who loses his fingers and job, swallows his pride and gets on welfare, a Puerto Rican teen who has no choice but to join the army, a suffering Chicana, a prostitute, a lonely old woman eating alone. The remembrances and vignettes rank among his best work. They are hard, deeply felt portraits of an unjust and cruel reality.

Similar qualities are found in the *Nosotros* materials of 1977. In two poems that he will later weave together as part of a chant which will become virtually his signature, the poet intones:

El fire hydrant	The fire hydrant
es mi playa	is my beach
bajo un calor	in a heat
que hasta desmaya	that makes even
las cucarachas	cockroaches
y los ratones	and rats faint
aqui en Chicago.	here in Chicago.

i

    am rican
      nigger/
        blanco/

                    indio/
                        in between
                            all which
                            is alive
                            good/bad.
                                when
                                    i
                                        was in
                                        darkness
                                        you
                                        turned
                                        me
                                        down.
                                    can i forgive
                                    you for that?
        i can.
        i
        am
        not
        like
        you.[8]

Some of the longer poems which follow are far from his best, but
one, "Tecata" (*Nosotros*, p. 4), gives us a harsh portrait of how
country Puerto Rican values are bludgeoned by the urban night-
mares which lead from drugs to death. And finally, in "Fame," we
have one of several run-on catalogue poems that are usually his
biggest successes:

    now that i have been discovered
    i will no longer write nasty poems about america.
    i will no longer hang her flag in the bathroom.
    i will no longer scream that the only good system
    is the chicago sewer system even though it clogs up at times...
    . . . .
    I will be discussed in english classes,
    the types of rhymes I used
    the deep-hidden meanings in my lines and

> how inspiration hit me in a chicago rain.
> (*Nosotros*, pp. 11-12).

In a much more recent poem, Hernández says, "I want to be a real poet/ so I can participate in poetry-discussions." Now that Hernández is more or less famous (at least in Chicago), here we are dissecting and assessing him. It's a hard operation to perform on so friendly and loving a poet. In a telling statement, he notes, "Being from Illinois and Chicago, the environment, the place of the city definitely influences the images and rhythm of poetry. . . . Being in a racist town," he adds, "Latino poets must be slicker, tougher, and no holds barred kill with kindness artists." In *Despertando* sometimes the situation leads to anger:

> I do not care who you
> are or why
> here is me from not the united states
> of amerikkka in
> chicago.
> dirt stench
> shit whores
> wiskey wine
> sweat piss time
> grass trees sky
> ("El Hispano" in *Despertando*, p. 52).

But the other side of this harsh attack is the sentimental, populist Hernández, who loves love, becomes gushy about the people, and virtually sinks his city rhythms in syrup. If love and truth are to win over a world of hatred and lies, let the victory be hard fought so that it has some genuine equivalency to the problems facing us in life. If David Hernández finds his way out of the dilemma of being "Chi-town brown" in the U.S. belly of the shark, if he never forgets that many of his brethren have not found their way, if those brethren are the real source and stuff of his work, could it be that in finding his way through writing, he has sometimes come to identify the writers or his white-Latin artist-art-consuming audience as his true brethern? "I come from a proud tribal-heritage of artists: The Word-Dealers," he intones to his (sometimes mainly

94   STUDIES IN ILLINOIS POETRY

white) audience today. And he thanks his audience for making his
performance and life work possible.

Has the bitterness in *Despertando* and Hernández's *Nosotros*
poems grown into complacence? Has Hernández mellowed too
much? That would seem to be the conclusion one could reach in
reading his little collection, *Satin-City Lullaby*.⁹ But the total effect
of a present-day performance with the Street Sounds belies any
negative or nagging impression (even some of the *Satin-City Lullaby* poems come off as better than they seem on paper). What
keeps his work alive is his irony and his humor – not his indulgent
sentimentalism, nor his anger, but that side of him that makes him
and his listeners laugh at pain and ugliness. In this respect, we
would do well to consider a perspective offered to us by Puerto
Rican scholar Frank Bonilla, in 1974:

> The dialectic of impotence and stubborn resistence, however covert
> and diffuse, is perceived as a grinding friction shredding individuals
> and social ties, but is denied any prospect of political resolution. We
> are, perhaps, developing a dangerous virtuosity in documenting the
> prostration, insecurity, ambivalence, and ideological bafflement
> within our ranks and assigning too little value to the contrary signs
> that point to a remarkable capacity for survival in a context of
> prolonged and radical ambiguity.¹⁰

With the Chicago Rican and *Nosotros* poets, we can perceive this
dialectic of impotence and stubborn resistance, as well as of hopes
and frustrations with respect to apocalyptic political solutions. In
their works, they show a growing virtuosity in documenting
Puerto Rican prostration, insecurity, etc. However, above all, in
their greatest achievements, they have also shown the ability to
point to the Puerto Rican capacity of survival, to make something
of their difficult situation and to find new means of growth. This
aspiration is present in many of the writers; but it is articulated
most directly by David Hernández, who not only describes the
aspiration, but at times realizes it. So, to take a symptomatic
instance: in one of his most disarming off-the-wall narrative poems
(one he does without accompaniment) he tells of how he is tempted
to rip-off a newspaper from a neighbor's doorstep, but chooses not

to do so, because he projects, step-by-step, how the act could lead to a bitterness that culminates in world nuclear holocaust. Without any overt Latino referent yet deeply rooted in Chicago lore, this poem speaks comically about an absurd, dread surreality in which one can take nothing for granted, in which uncalculating spontaneity has become impossible, and in which the worst things are ever-ready to happen. In such a world, the refuge of intimate love, the profession of such love in a poem, sentimentalism itself, become dangerous, unmodern, romantic, unhip and eminently non-Euro-American options. But they are the options chosen by this eminently Latino poet as he makes his way, twisting and turning through the years.

Early Chicago Mexican Poetry: MARCH and Abrazo

Even before the Puerto Rican awakening, of course, the larger Mexican/Chicano population of Illinois had been on the move. It is easy to overlook the fact that two of the poets and several of the artists featured in the *Nosotros* issue were Mexican; and above all, it is important to note that one of the graphic artists featured in *Nosotros* and indeed connected with *Revista Chicano-Riqueña* since its inception, José Gamiel González, was also the editor and graphic designer of *Abrazo* and the founder of that publication's sponsoring organization, MARCH. A Chicano artist and perhaps the key arts promoter in the Chicago-area and midwest Latino arts scene, González established MARCH to emphasize and promote Chicano and Mexican culture. Nevertheless, the second issue of the journal contained not only Matías's "Where are the Latin Poets?" but another poem of his, plus one by Puerto Rican poet Carmelo Romero, which also appear in the *Nosotros* collection; furthermore, these two poems deal with Latino/Black relations – the Romero poem specifically exploring the question of Latino/Black unity through a portrayal of Juan Tizol, a Puerto Rican hornman who played with Duke Ellington. The presence of these poems suggests linkages between the MARCH and *Nosotros* projects, which extended to questions beyond national identity to broader minority unities and affinities. The Black blues and jazz

world connected with salsa. But were there Mexican connections
as well? Were there important crossovers and nexos? Clearly there
would be, especially as Chicano mural art connected Mexican with
U.S. urban mural traditions, and as MARCH poets connected
with Black and Puerto Rican poet/performers.

It is important to remember that *Abrazo* and the organization
which sponsored it were initially more focused on the visual arts
and that poetry was seen only in relation to the arts. Probably
because of the linguistic problem, as well as lack of familiarity
with the publishing process, the visual arts developed more
quickly, and it is perhaps true to this day that visual expression
surpasses the written word. Thus, even more so than in the *Nosotros* issue, the specific place of poetry as an art form was conceived
as part of a broader cultural constellation. In this regard, as in
others, it is fitting that this collection, edited by a young fledgling
Chicago Chicano poet, Carlos Cumpián, and featuring poems by
three young women poets, Rina Rocha, Joy Sato, and Ana Castillo,
also has a poem by muralist Aurelio Díaz on the theme of Aztlán.
It also has an ample poem by a man who while better known for
his work as a graphic artist was also the veteran of Illinois Latino
poetry, a man who had been producing and publishing his poetry
on a consistent basis since the late 1950s. In an effort to trace the
roots and development of Illinois Chicano poetry we must start
with Carlos Cortez.

The Contribution of Carlos Cortez

Cortez was born in Milwaukee on August 13, 1923, the son of a
Mexican Indian father and a German mother. He moved to
Chicago in 1965, where he has been a fixture in Latino and overall
Chicago cultural life ever since, as a graphic artist and poet. Cortez's formal education as an artist was "very minimal, consisting
only of high school classes and a few night classes at local galleries"[11]; but the fact is that Cortez's artistic style, deriving from
the kind of cartoon work which made José Guadalupe Posada
famous in early 20th century Mexico, extends the grotesque gallows humor found in much Mexican art into the contemporary

Chicano/Latino world. While it is very probable that Cortez will be remembered more for his linocut and woodcut graphics than for his verse, he exhibits some of the same virtues and limitations in both media; and it may indeed be said that in some ways, Cortez translates radical Mexican traditions (including graphics) into populist verse. All of his works are part of his unique stance in the Chicano world as the most overt follower of the anarcho-syndicalist tradition which, in the hands of the Flores Magón brothers, was the most extreme force in the panorama of ideologies and orientations fundamental to the 1910 Mexican Revolution. He drew his initial radicalism from his parents, who were workingclass, poor, socially conscious, and artistic.

Cortez is not an example of an artist who finds politics but of one whose whole life orientation, then, would make art a means of political and humanistic communication. His graphics speak in a striking, direct manner, often helped out with words. Bold, cartoon-like images ridicule corruption and exploitation and hail the struggle against these forces. So too his many poems. "I write poetry because [it's] . . . another form of communication," he says. "The social forces of repression and the consequent forces of rebellion have long influenced my writing as well as [my] . . . other forms of expression." [12]

Indeed Cortez's initial experiences before and during the depression led to his joining the Industrial Workers of the World (IWW). An understanding of Cortez's view of the IWW or Wobblies is central to interpreting his poetry, as well as his contribution to Chicano and Latino cultural life through MARCH and the direct impact of his graphics and writing, especially since Cortez notes that the IWW was "the initial force motivating my expression, and participation in any other type of movements was but a logical extension of that." This is to say that in spite of clear continuities between Mexican radical traditions and Cortez's contributions, we might still conclude that his initial orientations were not specifically Latino, and that there's a way in which his Chicano/Latino, as well as his Indianist and other, perspectives are overlays on what is essentially a "Wobbly humanist populism." Cortez's

Mexican father was a singer and orator, but it was his German workingclass mother who wrote poetry.

While Cortez would sometimes use corrido and other Mexican forms, he would seem more at home with Indian storytelling patterns, blues and white folk forms. His Spanish is occasional, and not deeprooted. While his graphic mentor is Posada, his poetic models are not to be found in Mexico or in the U.S. Latino tradition, but rather in such communal and popular English-language bards as "Robbie Burns, Jack London, Robert Service, [and then] the early Wobbly poets and the Beat Generation . . . who were the ones that caused me to say, 'Hell, I can write shit like that too.'" Thus Cortez is an American anarchist poet, a soap box poet as he likes to call himself, with a strong counter cultural thrust rooted in a hostility toward big capital, but also toward any forces (including existing socialisms) which he sees as destructive to human cultures, human creativity, and human potentiality, as well as to relations among humans and between humans and the natural world. "All forms of literature of whatever ethnicity have influenced me," he writes, confirming this view.

> Because of my own background and the subsequent external consequences that have influenced my choice of identity, I have particular interest in Indian and Mestizo poetry, as well as any other group [which shares] similar attendant experiences . . . I do not consider myself "Latino," "Hispanic," "Herspanic" or whatever. I happen to be one who uses poetry as a means of expressing certain strong feelings; and had I been been born of different parents resulting in an entirely different frame of identification, I no doubt would still be expressing myself as strongly with whatever ethnic pride that I may have.

There is no doubt but that Cortez's Latin and Indian identifications must be considered in this light. But why is it that his art work seems more in the Mexican tradition than his poetry? Probably because it was easier to hold on to the visual world than the linguistic one, through the process of cultural syncretism. To be a writer in the U.S., even a marginal one, meant taking on what one could in language. And Cortez remains more distanced from his own verbal medium than he ever was from his drawing. Cortez's perspective is ultimately internationalist. And indeed there are references to many cultures – to Indian and Mexican above all, but many others. Within his Latin identification, there are references to things Puerto Rican (there's even a "Corrido Borricano" among his early works) and critical poems addressed to Fidel Castro. There are poems on undocumented workers, and on other dimensions of Mexican life, but what is most emphasized in his Latino/ Mexican field of references and what connects most fully with his IWW stance and his poetry is the Indian aspect of his Mexican identity.

Although, like many people from Mexico, Cortez's father came to work on the railroads, and while much of Cortez's identification is with his father's proletarian past, he also emphasizes, and perhaps exaggerates, his father's Indianness. He himself identifies with Spanish, Mestizo, and Indian dimensions of his roots, but it is the latter which most marks the ethnic quality of his work.

Cortez started realizing the Indian side of his identity in Sandstone Prison near Duluth, Minnesota, where he was incarcerated for pacifism during World War II. That Indian identity grows from his early, IWW poems to his more recent mature work. It is primarily from the stance of an invented role as an Indian sage that Cortez looks upon what the white bosses have done with Chicago, the Midwest, and the continent and what they are trying to do to the world. It is from the standpoint of this sage, then, that Carlos Cortez at times uses pen names – first, C. C. Redcloud (this at least as early as 1962) and later, Carlos Cortez Koyokuikatl (the "spirit name" given him by a Spanish and Nahuatl-speaking Indian in the early 1980s). And it is through this Indian identification that he bridges the gap from his Mexican father's world to a world where he himself is the elder and wiseman – the ironic, pithy, bemused, and rueful voice of Indians and Mexican mestizos who are witnesses to and victims of the White Man's manipulations of the earth.

Cortez began publishing his verses in the late 50s in the Wobbly newspaper, *The Industrial Worker* (hereafter, IW). There was a need for a cultural section, and Cortez became a prime contributer,

producing new topical material week after week, publishing for
the mainly non-Latino readership that the newspaper had. Interestingly enough, his earliest work draws most on the blues. The
first poem he published (September, 1958) was "Blues for a Bus-
driver."

> The driver
> takes a weary glance
> In the overhead mirror
> Seeing for the thousandth time
> His equally weary load
> Of wage slaves.

A month later, there would be "Late Evening Working Stiff
Blues," and sometime later, "City Central Blues," "Blues for a
Fisheater," "Outta Work Blues," "More Blues by C Red," and "3
AM Blues," just to mention a few. True, many of these blues don't
sound or feel much like blues, there's no keeping to the rhythm or
pattern, and like most of early Cortez, the work is very uneven,
with some lines that work or half-work and others that clunk along
as he makes one political point or another. Sometimes, though, he
keeps more or less to his rhythm and to his blues form, and gets
something better:

> Well it's a long time on the street
> And the rockin' chair money's all gone,
> It's a long, long time on the street
> And the rockin' chair money's all gone,
> I'm down to rollin' my own
> And pickin' butts off the lawn.
> "Outta Work Blues" (IW, Oct. 31, 1962)

Consistency of rhythm and form are obvious problems in Cortez's work; another problem is diction. Writing too fast, worrying
more about what than how he communicates, Cortez doesn't seem
to grapple enough with language. Words sometimes break suggested rhythms and tonal unity. Usually it's a big Latinate word that
sloshes against the gutsier ones and makes a bit of a mess. With his
longer poems, there's too much chance for Cortez to mess up and
lose all rhythmic and poetic continuity. The result is often a mass

of verse that doesn't work or only half works, with some decent
lines in a series of flattened out, broken up ones. At times the
broken rhythms or diction patterns are intentional, as he evokes
his Indian sage persona as counterposed to rhythms and norms
corresponding to urban modernity. And it is also true that among
his best poems are some relatively long ones. But Cortez is usually
most at home in fragments or in short, pithy forms, some of which
carry a punch line.

Studying Japanese culture (and having other Japanese contacts)
in the 1960s, Cortez wrote several haiku and haiku-like forms, and
some of them are pretty good at catching certain moments, or even
matters touching not only on politics but urban/rural and other
forms of cultural dissonance:

> Dawn merging
>   With a street light
>   At the bus stop;
>   Somewhere a rooster
>   Crows . . .
> ("Morning Haiku," IW, Sept. 11, 1963)

> Wise little pigeons
> they know
>   How to decorate
> The courthouse.
> ("Springtime Haiku," 4, IW, April 12, 1961)

And there are his little vignettes that express working class feelings:

> You with your million
>   evil green window
>   eyes,
> You swallow me every
>   evening;
> And puke me every
>   morning.
> . . . .
> Damn you.
> ("3rd Shift," IW, June 6, 1960)

Or ones about Chicago that give us a real sense of place:

> Winter morning
> The factory whistle
> Stabs the sky
> Like a knife.
> ("Windy City Haiku, 4", IW, Jan. 11, 1961)

> In a chilly alleyway
> Off West Madison Street,
> Santa Claus is an old man
> With a dirty beard
> Passing a bottle of cheap
> Muscatel
> To his buddies.
> ("Windy City Christmas," IW, Dec. 18, 1961)

Cortez has not been without a certain recognition as a popular workingclass writer. His "Outa Work Blues" was included in the IWW's *Little Red Song Book* and distributed to the more than fifty IWW chapters throughout the world; the poem was reprinted in Walter Lowenfels' *Poets of Today* (NY: International Publishers, 1964). His most comprehensive poem, the one which anticipates all the others, is his hymn to oppressed Indians, Mexicans, Swedish labor organizers, tyranized Jews, Haymarket Germans, brutalized U.S. and Caribbean blacks: "Where are the Voices?" First published for the 1960 May Day issue of *The Industrial Worker*, the poem later appeared in one of the major Chicano publications, *El Grito del Sol*, and then in the First Canto Al Pueblo Anthology. One of his most important expressions of Indian roots, "This is the Land," was his contribution to the 1979 issue of *Abrazo*, and it was reprinted in Scott, Foresman's high-school textbook, *The United States in Literature* (1979). Indeed, the Carlos Cortez Koyokuikatl who comes to his maturity in Chicago is a writer whose vision was already shaped in Milwaukee, and then is affected by and contributes to the emergent Chicano movement. His contribution to midwest and Illinois latinismo is in his radical internationalist vision, and also his characteristically slow-paced, ironic Indian voice which achieves a wry dissonance with urban rhythms, vocabulary, and norms.

> After days of cold rain;
> Thru the haze
> Peers the ghost of Tahoma.
> ("Seattle Haiku," IW, Dec. 4, 1963)

There is also a sexy erotic Carlos Cortez, but this Carlos is never separate from the Carlos who, starting in the early 60s, is taken by the contrast between the city and nature, who recreates Indian legends, who bemoans the smog and dirt, the acid rain, the radiation and fallout, the gradual extinction of species, and the racism and pretensions of his contemporaries, including those Latinos who attempt to deny their Indian or black blood. His growing critique encompasses all those who would destroy all that is worthy and creative in the world. This is the Carlos whose basic orientation was to influence his younger friends, Carlos Cumpián among them, and whose indigenist and anarchist radicalism and ecological anti-urbanism were to serve as essential parts of the Chicago Latino emergence.

Carlos Cumpián: Aztlán in Chicago

> Today I thought I'd call home
> so I got on the telephone
> and said, "Operator, please give me
> Aztlán person to person."
> She replied: "Sorry sir, still checking"
> after 2 minutes –
>   she asked me to spell it –
> So I did – A-Z-T-L-A-N
> She though I said ICELAND at first
> but after the spelling she said
> What?!! AZTLAN!
> She said is this some
> kind of a joke.
> I said, "No, you know where it is"
> She said – "Sir – I cannot take
>   this call, but

> if you wish I'll let
>   you talk to my supervisor – "
> I said, "Fine, put 'em on
>   I got time" –
> Well her supervisor got on the line –
> And I told her what
> I had said before
> all she could say was that was the first
> she ever heard about it – I said,
> "You'll hear more
> about it soon!" – and hung up – [13]

If any Chicago Chicano emerging in the 1970s tried to stress roots, bring together urban and rural, folk and modern, the Cortez perspective with the Hernández sound, the feel for local life along with mainstream and U.S. Latino literary trends, it was the young poet and editor, Carlos Cumpián. Born in San Antonio, Cumpián came to Chicago with his family at age 15 and early developed compulsive literary and political interests. He frequently tells about being shocked by the city's Black/White racial polarization, being confused about where Latinos fit in, being moved by Rev. Martin Luther King, Jr., and progressively veering in the direction of Black and counter cultural modes of life and art. Gradually coming to maturity, he read widely, identifying with the marginal poets, with DiPrima, Ginsberg, Bukowski, etc., but also with the rabble-rousing proto-rap groups like "The Last Poets" of New York, and finally, like Ken Serritos, with Chicago's David Hernández. "I'm a graduate of the David Hernández School of poetry," Cumpián has said more than once, referring mainly to Hernández's skill at oral-in-person delivery. But surely the Black current in his work is direct, and the Native American inflections (in orientation if not in tone) are mainly Cortez.

Most of Cumpián's early poetry evokes Chicano street sound, and almost all his work to date is profoundly and directly urban in its irony, cynicism, and sarcasm. But what modifies all of this is his strong ideological commitment to the indigenous strains of the national Chicano movement and culture, to the more rurally and folk-rooted anti-modern dimensions of Chicano writing. There is a strong "Greenpeace" and Chicago "New Age" current to Cumpián's work and thought (a concern with health food, ecology, etc.) that grew out of his early jobs and friendships and that inevitably led him as a young Chicano to champion indigenous pre-capitalist culture and to work closely with Jos González and Carlos Cortez in the development of MARCH. It is this unusual synchretism of New Age and Chicano indigenist ideology which generates contradiction and tension within the urban patter and verbal twists and turns that dominate his poetic style. It is also this element which, probably in homage to his pre-midwestern roots, enables him to tie his overt Chicago orientation to Chicano perspectives rooted in the deep Southwest.

Cumpián began publishing in the mid-70s, after joining MARCH and co-editing the literary section of the two issues of *Abrazo*. In 1977, he helped organize the first Canto Al Pueblo, an annual festival of Chicano/Latino arts and literature; and he participated increasingly in many Chicano cultural events in the Midwest and Southwest. Of all the workingclass Latino poets living in Chicago, he is probably the one who has read the most U.S. Latino literature, and literature in general, and the one who has done most to bring evolving national Latino themes and motifs into Chicago Latino writing. The youngest of the well-known first-wave Chicago Latino writers, he is the one nevertheless who rivals Hernández in his interaction with mainstream Chicago and Illinois writing circles. This role of linkage and the breadth of Cumpián's concerns lend a certain eclecticism to his opus. Themes of ecological destruction, genocide, empire-building, presidential bungling, the arms race, immigration raids, economic and racial discrimination, pre-capitalist or pre-colonial Indian mysticism, fashion, Chicago street crimes, Latin American wars of liberation, and perhaps above all cultural resistance, alternate as subjects of his poems. And Cumpián enjoys weaving his themes together. Like Hernández and Serritos, we are dealing with a poet most of whose early work has been oriented toward performance. Like them, he has written several poems which seem to be created through a series of improvised associations off a given motif, an extension from a prime frame of reference to the poet's most pressing preoccupations that are so linked, of course, that two, three, or any number of them often bubble forth in a single work. And this may put a strain on poetic structure in a traditional sense, and may seem to belie the impression he has made and maintained (one reiterated again and again by his commentators) of being notably direct and accessible.

A good instance of the standard perspective on Cumpián emerges in a news story by Josh Spaarbeck about one of the poet's presentations in 1986. Arguing for the "honest and directness" of Cumpián's poetry, as well as its openness to highly rhythmic and theatrical presentation, Spaarbeck notes:

> Much of Cumpián's poetry deals with social and political issues of the day. The problems in El Salvador and Nicaragua crop up often in his work, as does the plight of the American Indian. In addition, popular culture and advertising are often lampooned. But his work is generally as humorous as it is biting, and he is adept at drawing in his audience rather than putting them off.[14]

There is no question that audiences almost always enjoy Cumpián's work. But is he as accessible as he appears? The fact is that Cumpián's readings generate an atmosphere of shared assumptions and complicity. Listeners sometimes suspend disbelief, disagreement, and even comprehension for the sake of participating in the fun Cumpián generates. The result is that they often end up agreeing without understanding fully what they've heard or even knowing that's the case. And of course, since Cumpián believes part of his responsibility is to teach (and I would add, preach), he often is able to help his listeners actually "hear" things that they would not understand if they were to simply read the poem. Explanations and quips accompanying the poem are part of the performative process. But the major dimensions are tone and delivery. When he's on, who would not follow him and at least seek to believe what he believes?

Yet Cumpián is not so readily accessible after all. He puts greater demand on his readers than even his more sympathetic critics may claim. And perhaps there is a problem with his poems for those who have never watched him and lack the "histrionic sensibility" to imagine what the poems may be like in their true performative state. There are many who are unable to project through the written signs to the deeper structural and symbolic pattern which Cumpián has imbedded, and which can be grasped or intuited best through a hearing (along with tone shifts, quips, and more extended explanations) but which the reader may only get at through the most careful attention beyond the surface transparency of the text. These matters might be resolved for readers if we finally had a collection of his work, but lacking this, we generally get to enjoy his poems only through their success on the performative level, grasping what we can experience or imaginatively recreate.

The "Aztlán" reference is his poem "Cuento" may well be a case in point. No poem of Cumpián's could better and more simply sum up his goal as a writer and yet display the problem which his directness generates. For the fact is that over twenty years of Chicano ideological production are still not enough to enable one not versed in Chicano lore to grasp all the implications Cumpián ascribes to that lore's key mythic place. In this light and happy poem, the poet negotiates his way through our modern bureaucratic technocratic system in order to tell a representative of one of the system's main sub-divisions that the Chicano world is here, in Illinois as it is all over, that it is not strictly a geographic space, or a geo-political point of resistance to U.S. hi-tech domination. But what does Aztlán mean here to one who doesn't know? Here, precisely in a poem about Cumpián's core subject, Cumpián chooses not to elaborate his meaning. Instead, he truncates it, ends the poem where, one might say, meaning and true development should begin. Then, what is achieved by this procedure? It would seem to be nothing less than a calculated Brechtian effect by which the poet opens the door to several levels of interpretation, or misunderstanding. The key to all this is that we are dealing with a poet whose oral/performance orientation always leaps metonymically along an associative chain which extends beyond what is

structured into the text. In this light, the simplest explanation of
the "Cuento" poem is to say, "I'm not telling you what Aztlán is
because in your hierarchical system and discourse world I would
not be able to communicate it. It would take more than one poem,
more than one poet. It might take another world. And what if you
knew of Aztlán? We've lived among you for decades, but you've
never understood us. You should have known all along any way.
And as for our sacred space, it's older than your America. It's been
around for years, and you never noticed. But don't worry. Given
our growing presence, it'll ring loud and clear soon enough."

On this basis, I would argue, then, not that the poem is a failure
of under-elaboration, but rather a fine preface to Cumpián's opus
thus far. But to make my point more fully, I would have to enter
complex discussions, which would prove Cumpián's point (you'd
be hearing about Aztlán) but would simultaneously obviate the
notion of the poem's simplicity. Indeed, the resultant discourse
would probably end up being one of Cumpián's more typically
elongated verbal structures in which, in the process of exploring
the implications of Aztlán, still more complicatons would emerge.

Instead of entering into such a complicated approach to Cumpián, a better procedure would be to try to describe that underlying
consciously worked out structural grid which distinguishes his
efforts from those of the other metynomic city rappers. First, we
are dealing with a poet who, like his spiritual father, Carlos Cortez,
sees the world as a harmonious cycle disrupted by European con-
quest, gringo invasion, and all that which we call history. History
is in many respects the rapist, the enemy, but there is no uneating
the apple; once in the stream, one must swim or die. Cumpián
devours history, every aspect of what is to him a fallen world,
marking the stages, the dates, and modes of disintegration, promoting consciousness of further forces of destruction and creation,
filling in the missing pages, calling attention to false and illusory
modes of salvation, and above all, searching in Chicano and Native
American lore for all ways of recovering spiritual wholeness, all
ways of moving toward human regeneration. Some of the dates on
his world calendar are most obvious: 1492, 1521, 1848, and of

course 1945 (the Bomb). Many other dates can move to the fore-
ground: the date of Custer's Last Stand, the battle of Puebla in
1862, the U.S. attack on Veracruz in 1914, the Chicano moratorium
of 1970, etc. Countless other dates, events, issues, could be mentioned, because Cumpián's new poems usually mean filling in
another series of blanks in the macro-history of human destructiveness and resistance.

Through it all, through the mindspins of his many improvisa-
tions, the basic scenario remains his mythified history of the rape
of Indian land and being. The scenario enters in a city mural
project, as

> African/Spanish/Taino
> destinos . . . mix
> mambo y salsa realities
> we can dance today
> under our island and mainland
> star before the weather
> does a broken treaty number
> on us all . . .[15]

It is there as "el koca-kola symbol" dominates the sky in a tiny
Mexican town, and joins hands "with the/ ghost of Huitzilopochtli
in/ carrying away/ our teeth and rust." It is there in his references to
the coyote-shaman figure; in his references to "raza humiliation"
as a TV Colombian coffee picker is deported along with the entire
kitchen crew of a popular eatery; in his reference to "the curse of
Cain/ on our frozen lands." Scene after destructive scene appears
in poem after poem by Cumpián, but of course it's all there with
his sense of sarcasm and humor, as he looks for signs of rebirth,
hope.

And recently, the signs appear. For some of the comic rapping
litanies of woe on woe take on greater historical richness than ever
(e.g., his unpublished poem on Stalin, "Man of Steel"), and
perhaps more striking, we have an emergent turn to shorter forms
dealing with more intimate emotions and scenes, probably corresponding to his maturity and the influence of more varied poetic
forms and life modes. So, in "After Calling," a simple poem which

implicitly parallels "Cuento" and recalls us to the painful distances
generated by the Mexican diaspora, he writes of a telephone con-
versation with his grandmother living alone in San Antonio:

> In Chicago I hear
> her complaints
> and try to say
> the pain will go
> away
> before we have to
> hang up the phone.[16]

Next, he portrays the uncertainties of the human future in a poem
about his son: [17]

> I turn off my radio   after
> as the house settles   his third ice cream
> into winter darkness   and chocolate cake
> thinking of the night's   birthday –
> talk of nuclear   from his dream
> tensions after   I hear him cough
> billion dollar   then blurt out
> build ups   "I am Superman, Daddy"
> that would tear down   and in a moment
> global guardians   my Camilo slips
> under countless   back into sleep
> acres of a cold   to dream free of fear
> spinning cinder.   between the innocence
>   of the Lamb
> My other eyes   and the curse of Cain.
> are asleep in
> the bedroom
> of the Lamb

And, finally in one of his unpublished poems, he writes to mentor
Carlos Cortez of a new and fruitful compact with the midwest land
– some symbolic effort to redeem the Cain's curse: [18]

> After a long absence   winter and summer
> you wanted to see   father and mother
> the green sapling   . . . .
> planted in the yard   past and present

by the hands which	meeting in one flesh.
once carried you as a child.	
Standing under its	El arbolito
mature shade	still stands,
you and your bride to be	now a tree in Wisconsin
gathered around its	years after the planters
full trunk and	have gone,
embraced,	leaving a reminder
rain and sun	of what cario can mean.
soil and wind	

Still developing, finding his way through the maze of a changing world he always makes every effort to understand and confront with courage and humor, Cumpián will probably move on to new forms, new styles as he attempts to redeem the earth's violation and regenerate Aztlán, by planting a tree in the Midwest (in Chicago, Illinois, and the U.S.) that grows and reaches out its branches to all the long distances in the wide world beyond.

Final Remarks

As Chicago Latino poetry developed, other voices emerged which would add to the growing chorus and transform the music of Illinois poetry. The Casa Cultural Latina of the University of Illinois published a little book by Roberto Hernández, entitled *Yo el Latino/I the Latino* (Champaign: Casa Cultural Latina, 1975); and over the years, its *Literary Magazine* published some young poets. In 1977, Ricardo Mario Amézquita, born and raised in the small Chicano enclave in Sterling, Illinois, published a small volume, *Eating Stones*, in the Sangamon Poets Series. Besides Hernández, some of the Puerto Rican "Nosotros" writers, and above all, Salima Rivera, continued to publish.

Then new Mexican and Chicana female voices generated new poetic themes, styles, and forms. Women such as Marilou Castillo, Margerite Ortega, Emma Yolanda Galván, and Rina Rocha appeared. And then, the two most important Chicana writers, Ana Castillo and Sandra Cisneros, published their first work, only to move on to other places, the publication of their first books, and their growing fame as prime representatives of new Chicana feminism. Among the writers who stayed in Illinois, several represented new directions. Prolific poet Carmen Pursifull, of Puerto Rican and Spanish parents, began publishing poems that portrayed the Nuyorikan universe of the 1950s and her efforts to mesh her Latin roots with midwest circumstances. Meanwhile, several Puerto Rican radicals, sent to various prisons around the country, wrote poems about their plight and their aspirations. At least two of them, Luis Rosa and the gifted painter, Elizam Escobar, wrote poetry of some richness, under the influence of the late Puerto Rican revolutionary poet, Juan Antonio Corretjer.

Clearly, almost all the important new poets emerged in Chicago itself. Beatriz Badikian, a Greek Argentine poet, brought a distinctly hybrid South American-Mediterranean flavor to her writing; Achy Obejas, a highly inventive playwright and journalist as well as poet, brought middle-class Cuban and feminist lesbian currents as she explored the polarities of her identity in the U.S. and Chicago turf. Miriam Herrerra's writing also revealed the new kind of college-trained Mexicana poet. Margarita López Flores represented the tutelage of Cisneros and, indirectly, then, the impact of the Iowa writers school, even as she explored the problems of being a Mexican-Puerto Rican daughter of Chicago's barrio-world. Dianne Gómez, Carmen Abrego, and San Juanita Garza, three new Mexican writers, added their voices – the first two with frankly lesbian verse, and the last writer showing all the care and distance from ethnicity that one might expect from a student of Paul Hoover at Columbia College. Meanwhile, Ralph Cintrón, a Puerto Rican from the Chicano Texas valley, represented the first new major Boricua voice in Illinois, one which now reflected a broad literary reading in Spanish and English, and careful tutelage under Ralph Mills and other Chicago writers; and the most directly Mexican and proletarian of the new writers, Gregorio Huerta, began writing in English more than in Spanish and began drifting from his early romantic and declamatory base under the influence of Cisneros and his recent teacher Martha Vertreace. These and other developments are part of a process which implies a qualitative change of situation for Latino writers nationally as well as in Illinois. They have to do with the relative institutionalization and legitimization of Latino writing, and with the development of a somewhat firmer infrastructure in funding, instruction, publication, promotion, and distribution which enables the literature to reach a public and helps some of the writers to keep on writing.

As the careers of Castillo and Cisneros began to move, *Revista Chicano-Riqueña* left Gary for Houston. While the *Revista* continued to publish Illinois writing, it tended to select only what editor Nick Kanellos and his staff considered the best, up to the new national standards, so that beginning writers frequently had to look for other publications to make their first appearances. Helping to fill the void was *Ecos: A Latino Journal of People's Culture and Literature*, a modest student-staffed journal edited by poets Ralph Cintrón and then Carlos Cumpián at the University of Illinois at Chicago. It published Latino and Latino-related (e.g., black, Indian, Latin American, white dissident, etc.) literature, consciously declaring its intent to pick up the "Nosotros" project of presenting Chicago writers portraying dimensions of Chicago Latino life, in the hopes of participating in a cultural and sociopolitical Latino renaissance in relation to other struggles. Undoubtedly of greater distribution and impact was the journal *Third Woman*, edited by Norma Alarcón at the University of Indiana, and specifically dedicated to publishing materials by and about Latina women in their struggles to affirm and transform Latino culture and the role of women. Sandra Cisneros served on the board of both journals, and while clearly her contribution to the second was of greater national importance, her Chicago impact was felt rather clearly in both. Not only did she publish her own work in both journals, she also encouraged and promoted the work of other Chicago poets whom she came to know, respect, and sometimes teach. Co-directing a writing workshop called "City Songs" with Chicago black writer Reggie Young, she worked with participants López Flores, Badikian, Rivera, and Huerta, among others, to develop and refine poems that were soon to appear in

print, in the "City Songs" section of *Ecos, II*, 2 (Spring, 1983) and
other publications. The "City Songs" collection also included poems
by Herrera, Cintrón, and Obejas. The next issue of *Ecos* (Summer,
1985) included a poem by Italian/Mexican writer and editor Deborah
Pintonelli. Meanwhile, a glance at the issues of *Third Women* and
Revista Chicano-Riqueña (as well as the latter's namesake, *Américas*)
reveals several of the women mentioned above (Rivera, López
Flores, Pursiful, Obejas, Abrego), but also several new ones: Diana
Gómez, Linda Flores Quiones, Irene Campos Carr, Olga Ruiz Gib-
son, Grisel Valdes, Marisa Cant, and Miriam Cruz.

All this survey indicates that even as Carlos Morton, Ana Castillo,
and Sandra Cisneros left Chicago and Illinois, probably for good, to
shape their careers elsewhere, other writers have emerged, developed, and stayed on. But where are the Latin poets we examined
most closely? David Hernández goes on with his Street Sounds.
Carlos Cortez is still on the scene, and has given up smoking. Carlos
Cumpián is stepping up his own writing and poetry promotion
efforts. All three are still developing, transplanting their roots, and
taking off.

It may well be true that many of our best writers have generally
felt compelled to leave. And perhaps those who stay not only don't
get heard enough, but don't get the fullest chance to grow. A good
subject for debate. But at least now we have begun the process of
seriously looking at our poets, and perhaps we can soon evaluate
them, see where they are in relation to national Latino and non-
Latino trends and standards, and see where they can be expected to
go in the future. Wherever that may be in each case, we can be sure
that in Chicago, outstate, or elsewhere in the world, Illinois Latino
poets will appear, will develop, and will insist on being heard.

Notes

[1] Alfredo Matías, "Where Are the Latino Poets?" in *Nosotros: A Collection of
Latino Poetry and Graphics from Chicago*, a special issue of *Revista Chicano-Riqueña*,
Año V, No. 1 (Invierno, 1977), p. 37; and *Abrazo*, 2 (1979), p. 10.

2 For an analysis of the emergence of "Latino" as opposed to Puerto Rican or Mexican ethnic consciousness in Chicago, see Felix Padilla, *Latino Ethnic Consciousness: The Case of Mexican Americans and Puerto Ricans in Chicago* (Notre Dame, IN: University of Notre Dame Press, 1985). The fact that Matías's poem refers to "Latin" as opposed to "Latino" or "Hispanic" indicates how the poem anticipates future confusions and struggles with respect to the proper name for the broader collectivity. Clearly, this paper will insist on "Latino."

3 *Nosotros* issue of *Chicano-Riqueña*, Año V, No. 1 (Invierno, 1977), p. 1.

4 For a treatment of this period, see Felix Padilla, *Latino Ethnic Consciousness*, Chapter 2; also, Padilla, *Puerto Rican Chicago* (Notre Dame, IN: University of Notre Dame Press, 1987), pp. 117-143.

5 For example, he is the only Chicago Puerto Rican poet represented in *Herejes y mitificadores: Muestra de poesía puertorriqueña en los estados unidos*, ed. Efraín Barradas and Rafael Rodríguez (Río Piedras, Puerto Rico: Ediciones Huracán, 1980).

6 David Hernández, *Despertando* (Chicago, 1971). Friends helped Hernández type, reproduce, collate, and staple this volume of 60 pp.

7 Personal details about Hernández were provided by the poet in materials he drafted in February 1988.

8 Hernández, "Me la Buscáre" and "White Statue," in *Nosotros*, pp. 3-4.

9 *Satin-City Lullaby* was self-published by Hernández (Chicago, 1982).

10 Bonilla, "Beyond Survival: Por que Seguirémos Siendo Puertorriqueños," in *Puerto Rico and Puerto Ricans: Studies in History and Society*, ed. Adalberto López and James Petras (New York: John Wiley & Sons, 1974), p. 442. Cited in Padilla, *Puerto Rican Chicago*, p. 64.

11 Notes on Cortez in a 1977 art and poetry calendar published in MARCH, Inc.

12 These and other observations by Cortez come from his answers to my questionnaire, received in January 1988.

13 Carlos Cumpián, "Cuento," from *Caracol*, Vol. 3, no. 9 (May, 1977), p. 21; reprinted *Fiesta in Aztlán*, ed. Toni Enpringham (Santa Barbara, CA: Capra Press, 1981), P. 114.

14 Josh Spaarbeck, "Poetry Series Features Chicago's Cumpián," in *The South End* (Detroit, Wayne State University newspaper), October 16, 1986, p. 2.

15 Cumpián, "Muralist Incantation in *Literati Chicago*, Vol II, no. 2 (Summer, 1988).

16 Cumpián, "After Calling," in his book, *Coyote Sun* (forthcoming).

17 "Security," in *Coyote Sun*.

18 "El Arbolito," in *Coyote Sun*.

The Regionalist Tradition in Midwestern Poetry: Minor Leagues or Minor Key?

Robert Bray

Illinois Wesleyan University

> *Sorrow is/ a kind of order, loss a proposition/*
> *exaggerated by our faith in beginnings.*
>
> – Michael Anania, "Borrowed Music"

WHEN, now more than twenty years ago, Lucien Stryk put together *Heartland*, his enduring anthology of midwestern poetry, he professed no difficulty about defining the territory from which the gathered poems came. It was, he said, a "geopolitical unit" comprising Indiana and Illinois, Wisconsin and Minnesota, the Dakotas, Nebraska, Kansas, Iowa, and Missouri. In other words, the "Heartland" was, and is, like a great diamond in the middle of the nation, huge in extent, largely agricultural, continuous in its plains and cities on the plains. One could argue freely with Stryk about this grouping, for apparently he had taken down the atlas from the shelf and traced a somewhat arbitrary outline of the region.[1] But suppose that this is as good a "Midwest" as any other. Does it follow that there has been a distinctive poetic utterance across the heartland? Is there such a thing as *midwestern poetry*, created from recognizable natural and social materials, whose music registers the same to us, all the way from back home in Indiana to the first view of the western mountains?

To this extremely vexing question I would, with Stryk, answer yes. But to affirm regional utterance is immediately to go on the defensive. American literary history has usually either denied the existence of regionalism or ignored it as a sort of autistic literary sibling that never grew up and became national. At best, regional literature was said to be full of nature but lacking sufficient nurture. End of story, except for generations of noisy cranks and filio-pietists. Since the great nationalist surge of the 1850s, when it comes to literature "American" has meant eastern, urban, and cosmopolitan; "regional," western, rural, and populist. And this is true today: in the expanding universe of the literary canon, among the babble of special pleadings, scarcely any voice is heard suggesting that regional writers – in the Midwest as elsewhere, living and dead – deserve their niches and pedestals in whatever Escheresque pantheon we think we're building. No wonder that in the national arena of literary "valorization" few writers want to be labeled "regionalists." They see from history and feel professionally that it's a put-down, and has been for more than a hundred years.

I certainly don't want to repeat, for the Midwest, the arrogant cultural synedoche of eastern : American. The strain of regional poetry I wish to follow is simply one tradition among many, probably no longer the central piece in the cultural patchwork. The poetry I have in mind is not defined by any of the common characteristics of a region – geography, folkways, dialect, class, and ethnic lineage – though it may of course employ these as poetic means. Which leaves as essential, I suppose, a postromantic (but often doggedly anti-modern) "country of the mind" formed imaginatively out of the agricultural past. In common with so much British and American rural poetry, particularly romantic, the best poems of this tradition are lyrics. They tend to value place over history and the personal over the social; to notice the city apocalyptically if at all; and to personify the land tragically as a deeply shadowed garden with fallen tenants.

Given the triumph of modernism earlier in the century, given the indifference of American society toward rural qualities today, such poetry must seem almost irredeemably irrelevant. Yet relevance in poetry, as in critical argument, ought to be judged by, among other things, the ability of "strong particulars" to sustain a generalization (or a form). To poets like William Stafford, who is a leading spirit of the tradition I am invoking, regional relevance is everything, sourcing in "the deepest place we have," as in "Lake Chelan:"

      in this pool forms
    the model of our land, a lonely one,

> responsive to the wind. Everything we own
> has brought us here: from here we speak.

The regional standpoint is not always the firmest – "here" in this case is an archetype of Narcissus' delusive reflecting pool – but it is the deepest. In another familiar poem Stafford asks the earth a question and gets an answer embroidered around this maxim: "[H]ave a place, be what that place/ requires," implying no unique natural place but a world of wellsprings that we must tap for relevance, the earth whispering poets where these quick freshets are, the poets, like Calibans, showing us how we too may prosper – or not, depending on how we treat the land, which is too often cruelly or casually. (Stafford knows that what places require may be impossible, and we fail to "be" it: elsewhere he says to the prairie dogs whose place in Kansas he has left: "Little folded paws, judge me, I came away.") [2]

Though vague as to particulars, we could probably find Lake Chelan on some map somewhere, just as we can locate Michael Anania's "Ashland," from which vantage he scrupulously watched "The Sky at Ashland" (it's on a bend in the Platte near Omaha). The difference is that we'd be able to recognize Anania's more detailed "picture," using his poem as a "map." Were I looking for Lake Chelan, I'd start with the northern Rockies and work westward to the Pacific. But the point about such places is only loosely geographical and not at all "geopolitical" – if it were Anania would need to note poetically the rest stop along Interstate 80 where the highway crosses the Platte: a strong and particular feature of place. Not that Anania avoids the large details of urbanization or is socially unaware. (Decidedly to the contrary! Read his Omaha novel, *The Red Menace*, or indeed the anti-pastoral called "Interstate 80" from *Riversongs*, a poem "written" from inside a moving car, the postmodern vantage on the midwestern landscape.) Rather in "The Sky at Ashland" the landscape is natural, not cultural: a single implication of roads, one lonely image of farming ("gray silos"); the rest is a wild garden place whose "natural" literary genre is the pastoral. In this sense of regional relevance, as Stafford himself remarked, "Kansas is everywhere" (at least he said so according to Thomas McGrath who was quoting Robert Bly).[3] What Stafford brought out of Kansas he carried with him to Lake Chelan and points beyond: generic views of nature and "second nature" (I'll say what I mean by this below). All his "places" have proved portable and useful to his poetry, "wilderness" tabernacles for everywhere re-enacting the drama of place. This sounds "soft," I'll have to admit. But it's instructive to recall that no less hard-headed a poetic thinker than William Carlos Williams also defined culture as an enactment of place. He put it this way: "It [culture] isn't a thing: it's an act. . . . It is the realization of the qualities of a place in relation to the life which occupies it."[4]

So what then is "the regional"? *Je ne sais quoi*, he answers vaporously. Blame me more than the poetry! Alas, the situation's not much better on the other side of the title's colon: "minor leagues or minor key." I was remembering something John Woods wrote in the second volume of *Voyages to the Inland Sea*: "Strong particulars can carry a poem, even a career, quite far, but not out of the minors." By "strong particulars" Woods had in mind the litany of proper nouns and place names that adorn too many bad regionalist poems: "Gnawbone, Turkey Trot, Bean Blossom, Azuza, Climax: it's like living on a sparkler! Until you visit these metaphors. The Light in the East leads you to the opening of a Miracle Mart."[5] Woods' sarcasm targets "local color," a poor relation of regionalism and thoroughly discredited nowadays. Presumably, back near the turn of the century, when Riley and Guest and all that Hoosier rabble were busily versifying away, there was still an outside chance that turkeys trotted and beans blossomed all around them. Now the names are puns and games. But hold on: watch what a deft poet can form out of such dead matter. One of John Knoepfle's voices in *Poems from the Sangamon* is a prescient little girl, a "princess candidate sangamon county fair." She tells us she was "conceived/ far east . . . in indiana/ . . . the gnawed bone of my/ fathers desire the starlight/ of my mothers dreaming/ I am the bean blossom of their/ happy needfulness."[6]

For Knoepfle, the light in the east can lead to a county fair –
local, colorful. It's not *what* but how that what is handled.
Knoepfle's magical poem, whimsical and visionary together (the
whimsy, I would argue, lyrically serving the tragic), shows the
weakness of a major-league scout who arrives from the city with a
prior notion about "strong particulars." Why should *any* poetic
means or subject be proscribed before it is formed? Woods uses a
baseball analogy to categorize a crowd of (unnamed) lesser poets
and their poetry – good field, no hit, or something like that. But I
kept coming back to that one word, minors. Not *minor leagues*,
though this is clearly implied. What if Woods in spite of himself
meant "minors" as in tonality, key signature, registration? Then
not to get out of the minors would be vindication instead of
dismissal. A persistent vein of minor-key lyric runs through midwestern poetry. The poems I am bringing together, at least as I
hear and read them, powerfully connect with the hieratic tradition
of 19th-century British and American romantic lyric. Their poetic
effect is like Emily Dickinson's "heavenly hurt," felt, poignantly
and powerfully by turns, "where the meanings, are" in the long
shadows of her "certain Slant of light,/Winter afternoons. . . ." No,
she never made it out here (though traveling a good deal in
Amherst), but the last stanza is strikingly apposite to the Midwest:

> When it comes, the Landscape listens –
> Shadows – hold their breath –
> When it goes, 'tis like the Distance
> On the look of Death – [7]

These regional lyrics are poems of loss and silence, where what
is lost is both nature and second nature, and where silence offers a
quick opening for the poetic voice to sound back through time and
circumstance to an original, virginal existence. This originality,
whether edenic, graced, innocent, or only primitive and "real," is
always an object of transcendent desire – not facile but complex
nostalgia, whether a yearning for return or a craving for reality.
Loss of first nature – prairie and grove, the midwestern equivalent

of wilderness – has been a literary concern right from the moment of white penetration of the region and is related to national anxieties going back to the failed "Puritan moment" ca. 1620. "They" destroyed the land and the native cultures and "we" are guilty for it: aboriginal sin. The radical difference "out here" is that there's no place to hide and never has been. Thus the dominant aesthetic of aboriginal sin and the prairiescape is sublimity: awesome like the East, yes, but not so easily manageable in a picture or a poem as mountains, trees, rocks, and water. As early as 1827 Fenimore Cooper guessed what the prairies were like without himself coming West: He sent Natty Bumppo to the Nebraska plains to rage and die because everything east of there was already defiled, no fit place for a natural hero's apotheosis. Natty's Jeremiads against American rapacity are the first in a long and continuing literary line (see John Haines' "Things" below). Among turn-of-the-century American poets Edgar Lee Masters (who else?) felt the tragedy of aboriginal sin, saw it starkly and without the palliation of "inevitable" American empire. In "Black Hawk" Masters put the painful case against white Illinoisans like the outspoken lawyer-poet he was:

> The White men had Chief Black Hawk's land;
> But with the years it wasted, thinned,
> It blew away like sand,
> It mounted the wings of the wind,
> Leaving the once rich fields
> To the gulch, the gully, and the dusty ditch
> Where earth had been so rich. . . .

The tragedy is more the Sauk's, the Fox's, than ours; and Black Hawk is the tragic protagonist, another "natural hero" like Natty Bumppo, though crossed only by the whites and not himself. But Masters, characteristically, extends the folly and the fall to all, neither rationalized nor accepted. We buried Black Hawk "In the uniform that Andrew Jackson gave," stood him upright, holding the cane that had been a present from Henry Clay: "In life he had not any staff,/ In life his life was overborne/ By slaughter and the need of corn – / This is the Indian's, the world's sole epitaph."[8]

Compare Masters' dark retrospection with the report of an early poetic tourist, a "contemporary" to Black Hawk. On a horseback through the "Illinois Country" in June of 1832, riding northwest from Jacksonville toward Dixon, William Cullen Bryant, Knicker-bocker and Hudson River nature poet, found himself uncomfortably out in the open, in the midst of "boundless" prairies and on the fringes of the genocidal Black Hawk War. Once returned to the friendly confines of New York City, Bryant composed "The Prairies," a long blank verse extravaganza (extravagant for him anyway!) of 124 lines in four "movements." Despite being based on alien feelings from an alien place, or possibly because of this, "The Prairies" stands as perhaps Bryant's finest poem, one of a handful that has kept him alive as a poet. It is also one type of the prairie lyric, the magniloquent sublime, whose anti-type (epitomizing, beautiful) is Dickinson's "To make a prairie it takes clover and one bee." "The Prairies" broadly fantasizes the imminent transformation of American wilderness into American empire: Nature and the natural about to be fulfilled by history – or is it damned? Just what ground Bryant stood on, actually and figuratively, is hard to say, but let's speculate that he beheld his "vision" about midway enroute, which would have placed him in Tazewell county, the "fifteen mile prairie" he remembered crossing before reaching the Mackinaw River.[9] Climbing to the top of a little rise, Bryant paused to take in the prospect. We all *think* we know the familiar opening lines of the poem:

> These are the Gardens of the Desert, these
> The unshorn fields, boundless and beautiful,
> For which the speech of England has no name –
> The Prairies.

Bryant's romantic program demanded that he "find himself" in nature, which he duly does. But along the way he also hears rumors of war and talks to a number of the volunteers heading north, one of them Abraham Lincoln. Without this experience Bryant might never have shaped the impressive second section of the poem: his darker fancy of the ancient "Mound Builders" whose culture (my neutral word: Bryant would accept either "civil-

ization" or "empire" instead) was so brutally and utterly obliter-
ated, or so he thought, by the same "red men" who were now in
turn being driven down by the ever-advancing whites: "All is gone
– / All – save the piles of earth that hold their bones – / The
platforms where they worshipped unknown gods – ." Westward
the course of empire, etc. But would America be an exception to
the "law" of decline and fall?

I think Bryant was anxious about this, just as he was anxious
about being caught out in the open – about a sublime bolt from the
"tenderer blue" of the midwestern sky. Would you be surprised to
learn that the lines quoted above are not Bryant's original opening?
In the first book publication of "The Prairies" (Boston, 1834) line
three is entirely different:

> And fresh as the young earth, ere man had sinned – [10]

As early as 1817, when he was pulling himself out of an early
Calvinism (the "Thanatopsis" years), Bryant had put a similar
thought into "Inscription for the Entrance to a Wood:" "The
primal curse/ Fell, it is true, upon the unsinning earth,/ But not in
vengeance." "Inscription" is otherwise a mild Wordsworthian les-
son, characteristic of Bryant: "The calm shade/ Shall bring a
kindred calm, and the sweet breeze/ That makes the green leaves
dance, shall waft a balm/ To thy sick heart." In this context the
"primal curse" seems like a doctrinal concession, insignificant and
unavailing. But its impact in "The Prairies" is much greater. Why
Bryant, by 1832 the genial Unitarian and optimistic democrat, first
put the line in and then excised it is anyone's guess. But the
reference to Eden and the fall changes both the sense and the
key-note of the poem, especially when we consider the somber and
threnodic second section and the startled recognition of the ending
("And I am in the wilderness alone"). "Fresh as the young earth . . ."
seems to me a much better line; moreover, it has the effect of
making of the prairie garden a metaphor from the outset (man *has*
sinned; therefore even the best of first nature is *like* a paradise, the
poem at best a representation of an emblem) and intensifying the
aesthetic play between beauty and sublimity (Garden: Desert;

beautiful: boundless), slanting towards the sublime, as if a sudden cloud-shadow had cooled the ardor and darkened the eye of the poet. We too feel this minor shiver, and will feel it again with Bryant at the end of the poem:

> All at once
> A fresher wind sweeps by, and breaks my dream,
> And I am in the wilderness alone.

A few years after Bryant, Eliza Farnham, another New Yorker, would homestead in the same general area (Tazewell County) and begin setting down the life-notes that eventually became a remarkable book, *Life in Prairie Land* (1846). Here is her literary response to "first nature":

> I can never forget the thrill which the first unbounded view on a prairie gave me. I afterwards saw many more magnificent – many richer in all elements of beauty, many so extensive that this appeared a mere meadow beside them, but no other had the charm of this. I have looked upon it a thousand times since, and wished in my selfishness that it might remain unchanged, that neither buildings, fences, trees, nor living things should change its features while I live, that I might carry this first portrait of it unchanged to my grave. I see it now, its soft outline swelling against the clear eastern sky, its heaving surface pencilled with black and brown lines, its borders fringed with the naked trees.[11]

This passage has an interesting doubleness; it concerns both the prairie and the *view* of the prairie in writerly/painterly rendering utterly bleak and elemental, an evocation so completely opposed to the conventional picturesque that it cannot be readily humanized, nor would Farnham have it be *home*, only *hers*. Farnham's first prairie is (like Bryant's) "unbounded" and empty and undulant; but she reduces what she sees still further – naked, silent, dead; light and shade, the black and brown lines of winter afternoons. Perhaps the difference is difference in season, but in any case the temperature is cold. The landscape approaches a sublimity that Farnham both desires for herself and deems

essential to any *picture* of the place if not to the place itself. Hers is
a quiet and private vision – selfish – and the ancestor of much later
work which will seldom reach beyond the personal to the social
implications of what are, after all, absolutist standpoints. At the
same time Farnham's vision is heroic: don't touch it, America,
leave it (in Williams' words) "clean and aloof." [12]

No chance: the distance in time from first view to first cut was
an instant. By the late 1840s much of the prairie Bryant and
Farnham admired had been broken, cleared, and cultivated, initiating "second nature," the farmscape, what we are inexorably los-
ing in the final years of our century. Poetry calls this the last
essential left to lose, so we try circling back to firsts, attempting
recovery, as in Lisel Mueller's "First Snow in Lake County":

> All night it fell around us
> as if the sky had been sheared,
> its fleece dropping forever
> past our windows, until our room
> was as chaste as ursula's, where she lay
> and dreamed herself in heaven:
> and in the morning we saw
> that the vision had held, looked out
> on such a sight as we wish for
> all our lives:
> a thing, place, time
> untouched and uncorrupted,
> the world before we were here.
>
> Even the wind held its peace.
> And already, as our eyes
> hung on, hung on, we longed
> to make that patience bear
> our tracks, already our daughter
> put on her boots and screamed,
> and the dog jumped with the joy
> of splashing the white with yellow
> and digging through the snow
> to the scents and sounds below. [13]

Lisel Mueller is a latter-day German immigrant to "prairieland."
In Illinois she has become an in-migrant, probing second nature

for the residuum of the first. "First Snow" is consciously visionary ("and in the morning we saw/ that the vision had held"), like some of James Wright's best poems, and even reminiscent of Vachel Lindsay (in the lyrics, not the chants: for instance, the Blakean dream-vision "The Angel and the Clown:" "Where ragged ditches ran/ Now springs of Heaven began/ Celestial drink for man/ In Illinois"). I assume that the allusion to Ursula came with the poet out of Germany and adds to the poem both the theme of virginity and a mythic connection with Eden behind and heaven ahead – and their ultimate conjoining. This is all in the first section, of course. Then the vision collapses: daughter screams to break silence, dog pisses to stain whiteness, and "already" they "longed/ to make that patience bear/ our tracks": possession by imprint, bound to despoil. Only possession by dream can keep snow white: Mary Trimble's "October Snow":

> we knew it in
> the clouds rolling
> over in morning light
> like white snow in a blank
> sky covering our sleep
> like dreams of music we
> wake to the condition
> of music[14]

We desire "the world before we were here" because, from ignorance and folly and the will to possess, we don't belong where we are. Poems like "First Snow" assume blame for the loss of originality and look to the silences for a possibility of redemption. In *The Valley of Shadows* (1909) Francis Grierson marvelously summoned the "silences" that had animated preacher, poet and prophet in Lincoln's Sangamon country just before the Civil War. Listen to his evocation of deep nightime on the prairie:

> About midnight the stillness became an obsession. All Nature was steeped in an atmosphere of palpable quiet, teeming with dismal uncertainty and sombre forebodings. The flickering of a tallow candle added something ghostly to the room with its dark mahogany furniture, while every unfamiliar sound outside startled the mem-

bers of the family who were still awake. The doleful duets of the
katy-dids often came to a sudden stop, and during the hush it
seemed as if anything might happen. . . .[15]

Grierson, mystically distant from an Illinois he'd left fifty years
before, was far more optimistic about the "spiritualization" of the
prairie – of our sublime and apocalyptic cleansing – than the facts
of industrializing American warranted. Yet I recognize his "silences" in another striking poem by Lisel Mueller, "Cicadas":

> Always in unison, they are
> the rapt voice of silence,
>
> so singleminded I cannot tell
> if the sound is rich or thin,
>
> cannot tell even if it is sound,
> the high sustained note
>
> which gives to a summer field
> involved with the sun at noon
>
> a stillness as palpable
> as smoke and mildew,
>
> know only: when they are gone
> one scrubbed autumn day
>
> after the clean sweep
> of the bright, acrid season,
>
> what remains is a clearing of rest,
> of balance and attention
>
> but not the second skin,
> hot and close, of silence.[16]

Silence has changed meridians but remains "palpable," part of
the landscape until summer is gone and the music of silence lost
with it. "Cicadas" begins and ends with silence, word and condition, which helps me attend to the modal or minor music of these
poems. Not sound effects but form and tone, almost *formed tone*: a
sharp descent into melancholy, as in the last lines, an elegiac
quality heard and felt as modal – yes, reversions to the "still, sad
music of humanity," but sung "always in unison" ("so single-

minded:" Mueller leaves ambiguous whether the sentience is nature's or hers). Risking being silly, I'll say that I seem to hear a
kind of descending scale in the poem, the cicadas' song running
down, the same as I hear in my own backyard. And to begin again
they whine up like turbines starting (Dave Etter's "Cicadas"):

> After
> a long rain
>
> sun-stung
> cicadas
>
> with bright
> onion skin
>
> wings
> razor
>
> the heavy
> yellow air
>
> to wiry
> shrillness
>
> and red-eyed
> summer
>
> climbs
> back to love
>
> twanging
> ragtime[17]

Dave Etter is – and I say this with real affection for his work – a
c-major poet if ever there was one (though, as I've been reminded,
with blues riffs!).[18] So naturally his cicadas break the silence
"After/ a long rain" in a droning, "twanging ragtime," shrill not
still; their summer music rises to a high loud pitch and is sustained: Mueller's starting point for a long fall into silence.

I'm afraid I'm having trouble specifying what Heany calls "the
music of what happens." I associate it with tunes based on scales
rather than keys, I think of shape-note music and the "Sacred
Harp," I think of Charles Ives, I think of folk-songs that short-cut

history and plunge directly back to cultural time-zero. One mode
moves me most, the "Phrygian." Thomas Tallis, the Elizabethan
composer, used the Phrygian mode in the hymn tune that Ralph
Vaughn-Williams transformed so ecstatically in his "Fantasia."
Phrygian tunes move along the white-key notes of the scale, irre-
spective of half-tone dissonances. To those versed in the intricacies
of harmony, what I'm about to say will sound absurdly impres-
sionistic. Yet I'm convinced in my inarticulateness that modal
music produces emotions on the far sad end of the spectrum: from
the bittersweet moment or the melancholy sigh, shadowing into
the elegiac and finally the tragic. And something closely analogous
occurs widely in midwestern lyric – "plainsong" – often voiced
where we wouldn't expect it. In a Dave Etter small-town monologue, for example, where he plays one of those blues riffs. "The
Forgotten Graveyard" is an early, pre-Alliance poem, self-
consciously metaphorical and closer to Masters than Etter will
ever be again. Its speaker has a momentary "Spoon River" revul-
sion against his "townsmen" ("religious fakers, Republicans") and
takes refuge on cemetery hill. Up there, the usual anodyne of
"nature" – vestiges of first nature persist in country graveyards:
prairie relicts most importantly – almost works: "On this hill, the
clean smell of skunk." Nearby, "A woodpecker joyfully carves his
hole." And in the last line of the poem the place offers its boon:

> The sunset sweetens the mouth of a leaf.[19]

In Etter the sadness is generally as evanescent as the sunset; at
dusk his regular guy will gape and stretch, shrug, and go back
down the hill to town. But in many of James Hearst's poems the
conditions of tragedy are ineradicably of the land and necessarily a
part of the people:

> The clutter and ruck of the stubble publish the time
> That prompts my steps. I know what I have to do
> For my bread before frost locks the land against
> My hand, and fire shoulders the chimney flue.
>
> Rocks have a word that crows repeat over and over
> On the cold slopes of winter where the picking is poor.

It echoes in empty granaries and I learn by heart
To say in the hard days to come, endure, endure.

But now I straddle the field and break its back
In the vise of my plow, while a thresh of weather streams by
Sweeping up clouds and birds, leaves, banners of smoke;
I gouge out furrows, a starved wind ransacks the sky.[20]

The title of this poem is "Limited View," and certainly the perspective is: no expansive prairie landscape here but rather eyes to the furrow, straight and narrow, single-minded preparation for winter endurance. Melody and harmony are also limited, iambic rhythm broken by anapests, lines stumbling like the man struggling behind his plow over hardening earth. Long lines on the land, in the poem: eleven, twelve, thirteen, fourteen syllables crammed into ballad stanzas; difficult to read, nearly impossible to make music of.

But the music is there. What Hearst gains by a "limited view" is a solid center and a painful intensity. Nowhere am I more disturbed by this than in Hearst's "Landmark:"

The road wound back among the hills of mind
Rutted and worn, in a wagon with my father
Who wore a horsehide coat and knew the way
Toward home, I saw him and the tree together.

For me now fields are whirling in a wheel
And the spokes are many paths in all directions,
Each day I come to crossroads after dark,
No place to stay, no aunts, no close connections.

Calendars shed their leaves, mark down a time
When chrome danced brightly. The roadside tree is rotten,
I told a circling hawk, widen the gate
for the new machine, a landmark's soon forgotten.

You say the word, he mocked, I'm used to exile.
But the furrow's tongue never tells the harvest true,
When my engine saw redesigned the landscape
For a tractor's path, the stump bled what I knew.[21]

If I understand this extraordinary poem – more tragic than Frost,
to whom Hearst owes so much – it is about change, loss, and the
land's betrayal (not of us, but ours of it). Even the attempted
imaginative return to the Garden recoils tragically on the speaker,
like the speaker's "engine saw" striking embedded metal. The
cutting, abrading, harsh sound of the engine saw (so much more
monstrous than "chain saw") in wood: I hear the angular modal
music sawing up and down, back and forth over its confined scale
(quatrains again, the staff on which the rough-hewn iambs are
sung, five beats to the measure), but with no reconcilation at the
end, after the tree topples, no resolution. The landmark is gone,
the land marked, Cain is in exile. By the end of "Landmark" I'm
no longer hearing but feeling, viscerally: "the stump bled what I
knew" is a blow to the gut, the strongest I can remember taking
from a poem.

To be fair to Hearst, he does write lighter poetry. The sardonic
"Truth" underscores the inductive contact with the land and its
"things" by which we learn.

> How the devil do I know
> if there are rocks in your field,
> plow it and find out.
> If the plow strikes something
> harder than the earth, the point
> shatters at a sudden blow
> and the tractor jerks sidewise
> and dumps you off the seat –
> because the spring hitch
> isn't set to trip quickly enough
> and it never is – probably you hit a rock. That means
> the glacier emptied his pocket
> in your field as well as mine,
> but the connection with a thing
> is the only truth that I know of,
> so plow it.[22]

This is a one-sided Frostian colloquy with a thick neighbor, but it
ends with a motto close to Williams' "no ideas but in things."
Truth as connection with "things" is a grounded, tough-minded

intellectual stance, consistent with the overall "limited view." If there is a world-spirit, it's so inherent in the land, or so immanent in the mind, that no dualism is possible, not even an analytical separation for instructive purposes. Modern and monist. At the same time, however, Hearst shows us atavistically setting to work with engine saws to prove our otherness from that one. We could leave landmarks standing and benefit, but we rarely do. Hearst shoulders his share of the blame. Stoical acceptance of culpable loss – living down shame by doing the land's penance – is his way of meeting the tragic dilemma: "Rocks have a word the crows repeat over and over/ . . . endure, endure."

James Hearst's pieces have something of the old naturalism of Garland and Rolvaag in them, the poetry of broken backs. Longer poems of tragic loss forfeit Hearst's intensity (the modal tune itself) but gain the kind of rhetorical power found in Bryant (the "symphonic" perhaps, or Vaughn-Williams' elaborated fantasia on the modal motif). Thomas McGrath's "Poem" – unfortunately too long to quote in full – employs a four-movement form similar to "The Prairies," opening with displacement ("I don't belong in this century – who does?") and a recollected vision of the Garden ("In my time, summer came someplace in June – "), then modulating to a reiterated assertion of absolute, metaphysical loss:

> That was in the country –
> I don't mean *another* country, I mean in the *country*:
> And the country is lost. I don't mean just lost to *me*,
> Nor in the way of metaphorical lost – it's lost that way too –
> No; nor in no sort of special case: I mean
> *Lost.*[23]

More than a colossal blunder, this is the beginning of the end. "Someone had better be prepared for rage" (Frost warning!). And someone had better listen to the intolerable prophetic truth of John Haines' "Things:" "They tell us what we partly know,/ hidden by the noise we make:/ the land will not forgive us."[24] Once the lid is off, "things" pour out, the genius of place becomes an avenging jinn. The apocalyptic anger of "Poem" radicalizes even as it challenges Williams' "Raleigh was Right" (from *The Wedge,*

1944). To Williams' anti-romantic insistence that "We cannot go to
the country/ for the country will bring us no peace," McGrath
responds, yes, but through no fault of the country's: were it *there*
the country could still help. For Williams the country was yet the
country, but it didn't work; for McGrath, emphatically, the country is *Lost*.

"Poem's" second movement implicitly reveals why the country
is lost: because of the modern city, seen distantly and from on
high: "Now, down below, in the fire and stench, the city/ Is building its shell: elaborate levels of emptiness/ Like some sea-animal
building toward its extinction." The city is apocalyptic, "anti-
poetic." "[L]ong ago!/ long ago!" Williams mocks, "country
people/ would plow and sow with/ flowering minds and pockets/ at
ease – if ever this were true."[25] But if ever, certainly not now.
McGrath's "citizens" (in both senses: nationals and residents of a
city) are "unserious and full of virtue," beheld without love. Their
"rat's nest holds together," somehow – to McGrath a curious and
distracting fact. The city is a social joke in the third movement
(scherzo!), but not funny. So what to do, where and how to live?
Williams would make the best of it, making it the best (object).
But McGrath – and this is strange in view of his leftist politics, so
maybe McGrath's "speaker" is better – builds on the subjective:
the final section of "Poem" represents the personal as a final
bastion under seige, a pastoral enacted within the self, a walled
garden tended by a "talisman," a lover to whom the speaker prays,
asking only for everything that has been lost:

> Sun, moon, the four seasons,
> The true voice of the mountains. Now be
> (The city revolving in its empty shell,
> The night moving in from the East)
> – Be thou these things.[26]

Turning inward (involving) is the sanctioned lyrical way of recovering originality. James Wright's *Collected Poems* is headed by
"The Quest," an incandescent poem that leads the knight through
a wasteland back to his lover: not Eve in the Garden but the
Garden in Eve:

So, as you sleep, I seek your bed
And lay my careful, quiet ear
Among the nestings of your hair,
Against your tenuous, fragile head,
And hear the birds beneath your eyes
Stirring for birth, and know the world
Immeasurably alive and good,
Though bare as rifted paradise.[27]

Yes, this is romantic solipsism, one more form of possession, and liable to be the most tragically harmful in scarring its object. But Wright is full of "fits against the country"; he has wasted his life, the land is deserted. What else can he do?

Other poets have it easier, in easier poetry. When their loss results from "natural" rites of passage, as in Isabella Gardner's "West of Childhood," recompense is imaginatively easy. She re-creates beauty and grace through an Illinois child's garden of verses in which nature and her grandchildren may gambol: "That bud will leaf again, that choice bird sing, and paper boats sail down the robin days."[28] Similarly, in a poem called "Wheat," R. R. Cuscaden shows a couple "musty with love" lying in an apparently pre-lapsarian wheatfield. All of a sudden the machine is rampant in the garden: "A shower of cinders/ Draws you to me once again."[29] The "fall" is fortunate, the "Overland" express leading to more momentary passion, passing, after its moment of sublimity, out of the landscape into the weak nostalgia of memory. The wheat springs back, the lovers brush the cinders off and go home. There's nothing much wrong with this world.

Some of the most important recent lyrics have completely re-pudiated the 19th-century aesthetic of the "prairie sublime." To a mindful poet like Michael Anania, the sublimity of far-western American scenery is bogus, incapable of teaching us (sojourners in *le plat pais*) what we need to know. In "Missouri Among Rivers" (from his first collection *The Color of Dust*, 1970) Anania rejects what he calls the "violent picturesque":

I will not be led by complications of grandeur;
there is more to learn from the dull Platte,

> meager, cutting streams through sand bars,
> trees gathered about its banks,
> the prairies behind them.[30]

What should we look for in our own landscape? No "emblem or figured name," Missouri Among Rivers" concludes. Small particulars, then, that add up to . . . what? To a picture-puzzle of light and words that we try to work through time, or so Anania seems to be saying in one of his more recent poems, "On the Conditions of Place" (concluding section):

> As indistinct as water is in water,
> places dissolve into places, words
> among words, what is carried along,
> names whose sense shapes our memory,
> all that is said or might be said,
> Palatine or Platte, a leaf, a stem,
> a proper noun, a spit-curl of scum
> that draws along a moving stream
> the probable line of what is seen.[31]

"On the Conditions of Place" is one of three poems central to Anania's difficult and demanding landscape aesthetics/poetics in *The Sky at Ashland* (1986). The others are both considerably longer, the title poem and "Borrowed Music" (dedicated to Ralph Mills). Perhaps of the three "On the Conditions of Place" is the epitome:

> Sometimes it seems that more
> has been lost than ever remains,
> that we live in a slow passing
> among indecipherable signs.

Start with Williams' small particulars, facts with which to compose an object; end with reflections/refractions in the mind, languid impressions on a "moving stream," Stevens' intellectual reverie or Dickinson's lyrical (when particulars are few). The Platte "seen" from the Palatine and vice versa, "all that is said or might be said,/ Palatine or Platte:" portable places "carried along" in the mind, firm to begin ("names whose sense shapes our memory"), then softening over time and the river and finally dissolving:

"the probable line of what is seen."

The closer we look, the "better" we see? The poetic habit of close observation of homely, backyard nature becomes halluncinatory in the work of Ralph Mills, with a few of whose poems I want to end. But one last diversion first. Granted Anania's view that the midwestern landscape isn't sublime (but would he be happy with his own implication that our aesthetic is consciousness of dissolving and involving beauty?). Yet is it sublimity alone that produces "emblems and figures" in art? Surely another way is to people the landscape with representative humans (John Frederick Nims: "Man is the prominent fauna of our state/ . . . / delerious nature/ . . . Left . . ./ Conspicuous on our fields the shadow of man."[32]) and set them in action, for better or worse, creating emblems and figures that reconnect modern consciousness both with nature and the mythic past – and in their transactions provide relief for poets who might otherwise die of fulfillment, of taking everything in. I believe John Knoepfle *looks out* beautifully in "June Night on the River":

Tonight the river is
calm enough. A string of cars
drums along the Eads Bridge
toward Union Station.
Pullman windows charge the secret
spans of the bridge and tall
lights travel over the water.
They are hooded monks
gleaming among the piers.

Now I see whole mountains
honeycombed with monks,
and one of these, a boy
from Athos, fills the blue
Aegean with his own
image as he leans

beyond the prow of his skiff
and tries his luck
with a hooked line for his life,
his serious gesture.

The train goes its way,
the long lights go out. I pour myself
a careful beer, tilting
a cold glass above the Mississippi. It is
a lost river roiling
underneath the bridge. It came
from a deep cave on this
June night. And still it is
the one river Clemens
gave his own true Huck,
head buried in the black
knees of Jim, and the same
winds howl down streaks
of our summer storms.[33]

Knoepfle has acknowledged the influence of Thomas Merton. First Merton gave Knoepfle a subject, "an opening into my own region," but his "deepest effect" was a "sense of work as liturgy and liturgy as public work . . . that released my baroque mind. When I wrote about the river or of men laboring on the river . . . I felt that I was writing in my own tradition, and, finally, that this writing was in some way relevant to the present."[34] I imagine Merton in Kentucky at a singing convention, listening to hours and days of high whiny fa-so-la music and returning to his monk's closet to compose a folk liturgy. I can imagine John Knoepfle listening to Charles Ives' "Camp Meeting Symphony" and using the same folk modalities of lost and found and lost again in new poetry. Now I hear him reading, querulous incantation of many garrulous voices, some of them found but once found all his own: "I just want to say the country/ was in an agony of salvation."[35]

So at last Ralph Mills, close noticer. I am strangely drawn to his strange almanacal poetry – a shorthand of weather and plants that recalls the old diarist's "today some small showers of rain, some small spits of snow." As I read through the collection titled *Each Branch* the sense grows that Mills is looking for something lost that has made a big difference inside, where the meanings are. Anania's "indecipherable signs" or echoes of Eudora Welty's "when something is lost, everything is a sign." But Mills stares at certain things, ailanthus trees for instance, until he stares trough them, futilely, not quite getting the clues. Here is a "first snow" poem called "Cover":

> snow cover
> the first this
> winter
>   ice thatching
> bushes, raw glaze on the
> elm stumps/
>   nineteen
> years ago
> now
>   that day the ground was too
> frozen to dig
>   – and in July a
>   white stone
> flat with the grass

When that first snow starts to melt, as in "Brief Thaw," Mills sits "all afternoon in a light trance,/ a haze," hearing and "moving to a high-pitched music,/ the bell call/ of seeping drains." And in "A Narrow Space" some half-parenthetical "you" (the poetic interpolation is never closed) advises him:

> walk (you said
>   & keep
> to a narrow
> space
>   twisting rags of
>   memory
> into small tapers
>   that flame
> & die out

I will end with Mills' "Ailanthus, yes" because it haunts me and
arcs all the way back to Grierson's gorgeous Illinois Garden and
Farnham's reductive geometry of winter. Mills has noticed ailanthus now and again in *Each Branch* – "ailanthus," the tree of
heaven; and Grierson plays on *amaranth* – flower, color, symbol –
in *The Valley of Shadows* – "Amaranth," the heavenly flower that
never fades. Grierson opens a mystic portal back to the original;
Mills feels a nagging at his mind, bothering him, something he lost
and forgot he lost, a means of tying the ends together. He can't
help hearing "High-pitched music": beautiful, sublime, madden-
ing, deadly.

>   ailanthus, yes –
> & this window square
> blocked in gray/
>   unruly branches
> jab their hooked tips
>   at rain glazing them
> changing now back to
> snow –
>
>   not any dream, what
> she told me/
>   of having "lived
> long enough –
>   it's just how
> to know where
> you're going – "
>
>   even under clouds
> the wind
> dropping,
>   small banks, drifts
>   get lit/faintly
> blue at dark &
>   piled toward my yard's
> south margin,
>   its row of
> reddish boards
>   shoulder to shoulder with

cold-stiffened forsythia
leaning down – [36]

Notes

[1] Lucien Stryk, ed., *Heartland: Poets of the Midwest* (DeKalb: Northern Illinois University Press, 1967), p. ix. To midwesterners farther west the region might not include Illinois or Indiana or indeed any of the "Old Northwest," whose people in turn would probably reject the northern Great Plains and perhaps Missouri from membership. And to call *any* region of the United States today a "geopolitical unit" seems to me to ignore both the rather narrow self-interests of individual states and the general political and social homogeneity of the nation.

[2] William Stafford, "Lake Chelan," "In Response to a Question" and "Prairie Town," *Stories That Could Be True* (New York: Harper and Row, 1977), pp. 84, 75, 70.

[3] Thomas McGrath, interview with Mark Vinz, *Voyages to the Inland Sea*, 3, John Judson, ed. (La Crosse, Wisconsin: Center for Contemporary Poetry, 1973), pp. 36-37.

[4] Quoted in Denis Donoghue, "For a Redeeming Language," in *William Carlos Williams: a Collection of Critical Essays*, J. Hillis Miller, ed. (Englewood, NJ: Prentice-Hall, Inc., 1966), p. 126.

[5] John Woods, "The Region of Poetry," *Voyages to the Inland Sea*, 2, John Judson, ed. (La Crosse, Wisconsin: Center for Contemporary Poetry, 1972), p. 65.

[6] John Knoepfle, "princess candidate, sangamon county fair," *Poems from the Sangamon* (Urbana: University of Illinois Press, 1985), p. 95.

[7] Emily Dickinson, "There's a certain Slant of light," Thomas H. Johnson, ed., *The Poems of Emily Dickinson* (Cambridge: Harvard University Press, 1955), p. 185.

[8] Edgar Lee Masters, "Black Hawk," *The Sangamon* (Chicago and Urbana: the University of Illinois Press, Prairie State Books, 1988), pp. 38-43.

[9] Paul Angle, ed., *Prairie State* (Chicago: University of Chicago Press, 1968), p. 107. Bryant wrote an account of his journey in letters to his wife back in New York, including this revealing comment on prairie aesthetics, which could be a gloss on the poem he would soon compose: "I believe this to be the most salubrious, and I am sure it is the most fertile, country I ever saw; at the same time I do not think it beautiful. Some of the views, however, from the highest parts of the prairies are what, I have no doubt, some would call beautiful in the highest degree, the green heights and hollows and plains blend so softly and gently with one another" (p. 105).

[10] In the absence of evidence to the contrary, the common printing of "The Prairies" must stand as Bryant's "final intention" (copy-text). Yet two other versions of the opening deserve critical attention: the one with the differing third line cited

above ("As fresh as the young earth, ere man had sinned – ") which first appeared in William Cullen Bryant, *Poems* (Boston: Russell, Odiorne, and Metcalf, 1834), p. 39; and also the first *magazine* publication of the poem in *The Knickerbocker*, which alters the syntax in what apparently is an effort to combine the two other openings:

> These are the Gardens of the Desert, these
> For which the speech of England has no name –
> The boundless unshorn fields where lingers yet
> The beauty of the earth ere man had sinned –
> The Prairies.

This is the version that John Hallwas reprints in his *Illinois Literature: the Nineteenth Century* (Macomb, Illinois: Illinois Heritage Press, 1986), p. 68, on the grounds that the magazine text was itself widely reprinted in western newspapers.

[11] Eliza Farnham, *Life in Prairie Land*, John Hallwas, ed. (Urbana: University of Illinois Press, Prairie State Books, 1988), pp. 26-27. In his helpful introduction to the volume Hallwas locates the Farnham homestead in Groveland Township, Tazewell County (near the present town of Morton), and identifies the village they later lived in as Tremont (p. xvii).

[12] Quoted in Kenneth Burke, "William Carlos Williams: Two Judgments," in *William Carlos Williams: a Collection of Critical Essays*, p. 52. The entire thought is a complaint about Benjamin Franklin's tinkering: "To want to touch, not to wish anything to remain clean, aloof – comes always of a kind of timidity, from fear."

[13] Lisel Mueller, "First Snow in Lake County," *Heartland*, pp. 142-43.

[14] Mary Trimble, "October Snow," in *Prairie Voices: Poets of Illinois*, Lucien Stryk, ed. (Peoria: Spoon River Poetry Press, 1980), np.

[15] Francis Grierson, *The Valley of Shadows* (Boston: Houghton Mifflin Company, 1909), p. 38.

[16] Mueller, "Cicadas," *Heartland*, p. 145.

[17] Dave Etter, "Cicadas," *Selected Poems* (Peoria: Spoon River Poetry Press: 1987), p. 14.

[18] Thanks be to Peg Knoepfle, who, when I called Dave Etter a c-major poet, shouted "with blues riffs!" from the audience.

[19] Etter, "The Forgotten Graveyard," *Selected Poems*, p. 44.

[20] James Hearst, "Limited View," *Heartland*, p. 76.

[21] Hearst, "Landmark," *Heartland*, pp. 77-78.

[22] Hearst, "Truth," *Heartland*, p. 79.

[23] Thomas McGrath, "Poem," *Heartland*, pp. 125-26.

[24] John Haines, "Things," *In a Dusty Light* (Port Townsend, Washington: the Graywolf Press, 1977), p. 22.

[25] William Carlos Williams, "Raleigh was Right," *Collected Poems*, 2 (New Directions, 1988), p. 85.

26 The intended line space between sections three and four of "Poem" is omitted from *Heartland* but included in the version printed in *Voyages to the Inland Sea*, 3, p. 61.

27 James Wright, "The Quest," *Collected Poems* (Middletown, Connecticut: Wesleyan University Press, 1972), p. 3.

28 Isabella Gardner, "West of Childhood," *Heartland*, p. 66.

29 R. R. Cuscaden, "Wheat," *Heartland*, pp. 35-36.

30 Michael Anania, "Missouri Among Rivers," *The Color of Dust* (Chicago: the Swallow Press, 1970), p. 7.

31 Michael Anania, "On the Conditions of Place," *The Sky at Ashland* (Mt. Kisco, NY: Moyer Bell Limited, 1986), pp. 13-14.

32 John F. Nims, "Midwest," *Heartland*, p. 150.

33 John Knoepfle, "June Night on the River," *Heartland*, pp. 99-100.

34 Knoepfle, "Poetry in the Fifties: a Personal View," *Voyages to the Inland Sea*, 1, John Judson, ed. (La Crosse, Wisconsin: Center for Contemporary Poetry, 1971), pp. 31-32.

35 Knoepfle, "circuit preacher, lines after Cartwright," *Poems from the Sangamon*, p. 17

36 Ralph J. Mills, Jr., "Cover," "Brief Thaw," "A Narrow Space" and "Ailanthus, yes," *Each Branch* (Peoria: Spoon River Poetry Press, 1986), pp. 65, 48, 70, 105.